Soft Tissue Arthritis

Bursitis, Fibromyalgia;
Fibromyositis;
Fibrositis;
Rheumatism
Bursitis
Tendinitis
Rotator Cuff
Myofascial Pain
Carpal Tunnel Syndrome
Tennis Elbow
Golfer's Elbow
Tenosynovitis
Plantar Fascitis
and more!

by
Anthony di Fabio and Paul Jaconello, M.D.

Certificate

A prior edition was copyrighted in 1998.
by Anthony di Fabio, M.A. & Paul Jaconello, M.D.

Published by
The Arthritis Trust of America
7111 Sweetgum Road
Fairview, TN 37062-9384
http://www.arthritistrust.org

What Is Soft Tissue Arthritis?

First let me explain about the main categories of arthritis. These are Rheumatoid Disease, Osteoarthritis and Gouty Arthritis.

Rheumatoid Disease is one of those strange classifications that seem to cover everything including the kitchen sink. There are about 100 different names for Rheumatoid Disease. These are well covered -- that is the systemic nature of Rheumatoid Disease -- is well covered in our book *Arthritis: Osteoarthritis and Rheumatoid Disease Including Rheumatoid Arthritis* that you'll find on Amazon.com.

Osteoarthritis is also explained in the above book. Plainly Osteoarthritis is primarily a function of insufficient movement of the joints. When you were a child you daily ran and jumped and played physically so that your blood was squeezed into and out of the cartiledge at the joints, thus nourishing the joints. Normally children don't suffer from Osteoarthritis.

Gouty Arthritis is known by those sharp needle-like pains chiefly in the toes. The proper medicine and diet will eliminate gout in your life. The above referenced book will also explain what you must do if you suffer from Gout.

One of the common misconceptions that must be overcome to understand the above three categories of arthritis as well as soft tissue arthritis is that it is not true that whenever a joint aches, one has arthritis. That's the layman's term for the pain and its location.

So, OK! What is soft tissue arthritis?

Traditional medicine will argue that "arthritis" means inflammation in the joint itself. This narrow definition has never resulted in outright cures, whereas the idea that Rheumatoid Arthritis is primarily a systemic disease and that the joints may be but one place where the disease manifests has resulted in many cures based on the protocols described by The Arthritis Trust of America. So, what follows are categories of soft tissue arthritis as recognized and described in traditional medicine. Some of these named problems may be a reflection of what the Arthritis Trust of America calls Systemic Rheumatoid Disease, and some may not be -- but whatever the case, there are excellent treatments that will solve most.

Bursitis

When there's pain, swelling and inflammation in the tissues and structures around a joint it's called bursitis or tendinitis Such a condition is often called a "syndrome." These syndromes are very common.

The factors that cause or contribute to bursitis or tendinitis are: overuse or injury to the joint areas through play or work, bad posture, a poorly positioned joint or bone that causes unusual stress and other diseases or conditions.

Pain in the upper shoulder or upper third of the arm and/or severe pain on moving the shoulder are primary symptoms of Bursitis.

Types of Bursitis

There's a small sac which gets inflamed or irritated located between a bone This sac, or bursa, permits smooth gliding between varoious bodily structures. The bursa allows smooth gliding between these structures. There can be pain in the upper shoulder or upper third of the arm and severe pain when the shoulder is moved.

Trochanteric Bursitis

There's a prominent bone at the hip which has over it a bursa called the trochanteric bursa. Most affected by bursitis at this location are middle-aged to older folks and women. Walking abnormally can cause the problem. Symptoms can appear when sleeping on the side of the pain or upon arising from a deep chair, or from sitting in a car or climbing stairs.

Ischial Bursitis

Below the bone in your buttock is the bursa called the ischium. This bursa can become inflamed from being injured or from sitting on a hard surface. Ischial bursitis has been called "weaver's bottom" or "tailor's seat." Symptoms may appear when sitting or lying down. Pain can travel to the back from the thigh.

Olecranon Bursitis

At the tip of the elbow is a small sac which can be injured by gout, rheumatoid arthritis, infection, or a long period of leaning on the elbows. Swelling, redness and pain at the tip of the elbow are its symptoms.

Prepatellar Bursitis

Beneath the skin and in front of the kneecap is the prepatellar bursa. It may become inflamed as a result of infection, injury, gout, or repeated irritation from kneeling. Sometimes this is called "clergyman's knees."

Pes Anserinus Bursitis

The Pes Anserimus bursa This bursa is located just beneath the knee on the inner part of the leg. Jogging, over-weight or osteoarthritis can cause inflammation of this bursa. There is pain on the side of the knee or when climbing stairs and pain that seems to travel to the back and inside of the thigh.

Retrocalcaneal Bursitis

The Retrocalcaneal bursa is located at the back of the heel. Ankylosing Spondylitis or Rheumatoid Disease or even the wearing of shoes of the wrong size can cause painful swelling bursitis in back of the heal.

Calcaneal Bursitis

Heel spurs, excess weight, injury and improper sized shoes can cause inflammation of this bursa located at the sole or bottom of the heel.

Types of Tendinitis

Tendons hold the structure of the body together and are the portion of the anatomy that powers our muscles as it attaches to bone and muscle.

Rotator Cuff Tendinitis and Impingement Syndrome

The four rotator cuff.muscles move the shoulder away from the side of the body and turn it inward and outward. When there's shoulder injury or overuse of muscles, rotator cuff tendinitis. When tendons are pinched between structures that are involved in shoulder motion the symptoms could include sudden, severe pain in the upper shoulder or upper third of the arm; aching in the shoulder region; difficulty sleeping on the shoulder; or pain when lifting the arm overhead.

Bicipital Tendinitis

Overuse or injury of the biceps tendon located in the front of the shoulder typically causes inflammation in the tendon.Pain in the front or the side of the shoulder can travel down to the elbow and forearm.

DeQuervain's Tendinitis

This tendinitis is caused by overuse of the thumb tendons, such as by repeated pinching with the thumb while moving the wrist. Writing, gardening, or fine handiwork might be the source.

Achilles Tendinitis

Attaching the calf muscle to the heel is the Achilles Tendons which lifts the heel off the ground. Sports injury or improperly fitted shoes can be the source of the problem. One has ankle stiffness and pain and swelling in back of the ankle.

<u>Other Types of Soft Tissue Rheumatic Syndromes</u>
Myofascial Pain

In the back, neck and shoulders one can feel pain in the muscles, called Myofascial pain. When pressed with, say, the thumb one feels tender, hard points called "trigger points." It's a dull, aching pain which is located in connective tissue, the faschia. It can also be felt in the lower back and buttocks. Back strain or minor injuries might be it's source. Besides minor injuries or strains it could be associated with degenerative back problems.

Carpal tunnel syndrome

Carpal tunnel syndrome is a well known problem. It stems from the median nerve that passes between the wrist bones and a strong ligament on the bottom of the wrist which may be compressed. The first three fingers and part of the ring finger are involved. Carpal tunnel syndrome may come from injury through repetitive use or overuse, diabetes, thyroid disease, infection, pregnancy, or from rheumatoid arthritis as well as other types of inflammatory arthritis. When the wrist is flexed for a long time there can be numbness or tingling in the hand, and also often the feeling of a swollen hand and weakness of thumb upon pinching. The tarsal tunnel syndrome is a similar condition which can affect the nerve located in the inner part of the ankle that supplies sensation to the toes and the sole of the foot. Compression on the nerve at the ankle can occur with ankle fractures, rheumatoid arthritis, or foot deformities. A burning feeling of the foot can be painful.

Tennis Elbow (Lateral Epicondylitis)

Everyone has heard of Tennis Elbow which is pain in the lateral epicondyle where muscles of the forearm attach to the outside bone of the elbow. When the muscles have been overused like in sports, or as in tennis where a particular rotation and extension of the wrist and hand are called upon repeatedly one can suffer this condition.Gardening, using tools, or clenching your hand for a long time may also cause epicondylitis. The aching of pain on the outside of the elbow travels down the forearm causing pain with handshakes, finger movements and wrist motions.

Golfer's Elbow (Medial Epicondylitis)

Overusing muscles that clench the fingers cause a similar condition called Golfer's Elbow.

Tenosynovitis

Stenosing tenosynovitis results from a thickening of the lining around the tendons of the fingers. This is sometimes called "trigger finger." A finger can lock in a painful, bent position but can be straightened out with the other hand. There's tenderness, swelling and small bumps in the palm of the hand and also aching in the middle joint of the affected finger.

Plantar Fasciitis

Thickened fibrous tissue that spans the sole of the foot from heel to toes makes up the plantar fascia. Prolonged standing, running, heel spurs, flat feet, excessive weight can cause stress on the fascia which then causes pain in the foot.

Traditional Treatment and Prevention

Most traditional treatment is palliative, meaning that only symptoms are treated, usually with pain killing drugs or by the use of rest, splints, heat and cold application, physical therapy, or occupational therapy.

While we can't guarantee to cure everyone, we believe that there's numerous treatments that will solve the causation of many so-called soft tissue arthritis problems. For example, some of those we've described mention that rheumatoid arthritis could be the cause of a particular soft tissue arthritis. If so, then the solution is described in our book *Arthritis: Osteoarthritis and Rheumatoid Disease Including Rheumatoid Arthritis* found on Amazon.com.

Diabetes was mentioned as a causative agent in one form of soft tissue arthritis. If so, then see the solution to Diabetes II in our *Absolutely Phenomonal Medical Treatments* book on Amazon.com. It has long been known by caring doctors that Diabetes II is caused by a food allergies and this is easily handled. If it is Diabetes I, then see our book *The Magic of Magnetic Healing* by Dr. William Philpott, also on Amazon.com.

The above books will go into more detail as to how to get permanent relief.

The reader's main problem may be to find health professionals who are knowledgeable and trained in some of these procedures. If dedicated to wellness than you might have to travel to the right doctor.

Meanwhile, here's what we know and advise for the treatment of Soft Tissue Arthritis!

The Case of Maryanne Anderson

John Marion Ellis, M.D. considered his first proof of the value of vitamin B[6] injections to be that of thirty-seven-year-old African-American Maryanne Anderson, who weighed 195 pounds and was eight months pregnant.

Maryanne suffered from severe tingling in both arms and hands, together with severe swelling of her hands and feet.

Dr. Ellis reported that from behind his desk, "I was able to see that the tops of her feet were swollen so badly, the skin looked like the shiny rubber on an over-inflated balloon. I walked over to her, knelt down and pressed my finger into the swollen flesh. After I removed the pressure, the outline of my finger remained for several seconds in her bloated arches. This was severe water retention."

At night she experienced severe cramps in the backs of her legs, between her knees and in her ankles, and she'd had to buy larger shoes to accomodate her swollen feet. She'd had to rest constantly each day, and any time she lay down, her hands would tingle and become numb up to the elbows.

Dr. Ellis felt that her symptoms reflected more than the simple swelling of pregnancy.

Maryanne Anderson was treated with 50 milligrams of pyridoxine hydro-chloride every two days for a two-week period, and the results came swiftly.

Within four days Maryanne had skin on the top of her feet that were wrinkled, pliable and loose. Her oversize shoes slipped from her feet. Dr. Ellis was able to pinch flesh between his finger and thumb, and Maryanne reported less tingling in her hands and feet.

What are These Diseases?

Kate Lorig, R.N., Dr.P.H., and James F. Fries, M.D., report that "Most of the problems we tend to call arthritis don't involve the joints and really aren't even diseases. . . . There are a lot of names for these conditions — Bursitis, low back strain, sciatica, metatarsalgia, Achilles Tendinitis, heel-spur syndrome, sprained ankle, cervical neck strain, frozen shoulder, tennis elbow, housemaid's knee, Carpal-Tunnel Syndrome, and others. People call all of these "bursitis,' while doctors have fancier names for them. But they are all local conditions and are approached the same way. At first you don't even need a doctor for them, but if they don't respond after six weeks of self-treatment or seem alarmingly severe, be sure to see a doctor."

Symptoms are: fatigue, inflammation of muscle tissues; muscle weakness; pain, local tenderness, and stiffness of joints, muscles, joint capsules and adjacent structures; limitation of motion at joints; joint swelling and redness.

A group of common illnesses, whose source of pain is poorly identified in the muscles, are called Fibromyalgia, Fibromyositis, or Fibrositis.

Fibrositis, like Fibromyositis, describes inflammation of the fibrous connective tissue components of muscles, joints, tendons, ligaments, and other "white" connective tissues.

Paul Davidson, M.D., formerly Associate Clinical Professor of Medicine at the University of California Medical Center, described disorders that affect tendons, joint capsules, ligaments, fascias, bursas, cartilages and muscles as "soft-tissue rheumatism," and distinguished these conditions from "arthritis" which affects hard tissues.

Various combinations of Bursitis, Fibromyalgia, Fibrositis and Fibromyositis may occur together as "simple Rheumatism," known as recurring (Palindromic) Rheumatism.

Warren Levin, M.D. of New York City, New York, says, "Unfortunately, the term 'Rheumatism' is not very discriminating, as it is often used to include both hard tissue and soft tissue arthritis."

Bursitis is acute or chronic inflammation of a bursa, the saclike cavity with fluid that surrounds the location where tendons pass over bony prominences, or between tendons, muscles, and bones. Their purpose is to promote the movement of tissue gliding.

With Fibromyalgia, Fibromyositis, and Fibrositis, any body part having fibromuscular tissue may be involved, but the most frequently seen are low back (Lumbago), neck (Torticollis), shoulders, thorax (Pleurodynia), and thighs (Leg Aches or "Charleyhorses").

"Torticollis" is tonic or intermittent spasm of the neck muscles causing rotation and tilting of the head.

Fibrositis pains can be brought on or intensified by trauma, exposure to dampness and cold, and by rheumatic problems.

Distribution of Fibromyalgia

Leon Chaitow, D.O.,[8] England, reports that "Many children are now being diagnosed as having this condition. It often starts with flu-like symptoms and then becomes chronic, with sleep disturbance as a major feature.

"Fibromyalgia is now the commonest disorder seen by rheumatologists after Osteoarthritis and Rheumatoid Arthritis.

"Dr. Don Goldenberg, Chief of Rheumatology at Newton-Wellesley Hospital and Professor of Medicine at Tufts University School of Medicine, esti-

8

mates that there are between 3 and 6 million Americans affected by Fibromyalgia, mainly between the ages of 26 and 35 and with the vast majority being women (86% females against 14% males according to many surveys). Some estimates have the figures in the United States as high as 12-15 million."[41]

"Based on population size and surveys we can therefore estimate that between 750,000 and 1.5 million people in Britain also have Fibromyalgia.

"According to Professor Bruce Rothschild of Northeast Ohio Universities College of Medicine, nearly 25% of patients seen at rheumatology clinics are actually suffering from Fibromyalgia."[8]

Clinical Symptoms for Fibromyalgia

Most often a patient (usually female) will complain of fatigue, widespread pain and stiffness. Lacking better guidelines or professional knowledge, physicians may have already wrongly labeled this patient as being a hypochondriac, or suffering from a psychogenic rheumatism. According to data uncovered by a Fibromyalgia support group established by David and Margy Squires, Phoenix, Arizona, "the average person with Fibromyalgia has gone 10 years before being correctly diagnosed, seen 12 doctors, tried 15-18 medications, and were put through unnecessary operations for symptoms related to Fibromyalgia. On average 60% are disabled and unable to work, and 35% have had other members of their families diagnosed with Fibroymyalgia."[24]

Somewhat better informed physicians may have labeled the problem as (a) a connective tissue disease, (b) chest pain (costrochondritis or Tietze's syndrome), (c) tennis elbow, (d) shoulder Bursitis, (e) pain at either of two bony processes below the neck of the femur (trochanteric bursitis), or (f) back pain.

Laboratory tests will be negative. There will be reports of some sleep disturbance, such as repeated awakenings and also greater fatigue on arising in the morning than when retiring.

There may also be complaints of depression, migraine headaches, irritable bowel and pain in the temple and lower jaw (temporomandibular).

The diagnosis of fibromyalgia (sometimes also called Fibromyalgia Syndrome, or FMS) is confirmed by noting through physical examination a multiple of symmetrically located tender points called "trigger points." Their are 18 trigger points defined by the American College of Rheumatologists and eleven of these 18 trigger points must be tender on application of mild pressure to allow for an "official" diagnosis of Fibromyalgia. Eight points are behind the neck and upper back; four are symmetrically arranged, two at each side of the buttocks; two of them, one at each elbow; two, one each at the inside of each knee, and two at the sternum below the chin.

Fibromyalgic tenderness is often distinguished from normal tenderness by

9

an exaggerated emotional response, including crying, a withdrawal of the tender part of the body, and a worsening of the pain from days to weeks after the physical examination. Additional examination may then reveal added tender spots that were not noted in the first examination.

According to Leon Chaitow, D.O.,[8] England, almost 100% of those suffering from Fibromyalgia have muscular pain, aching and/or stiffness (especially in the morning), fatigue, badly disturbed sleep, and symptoms that are usually worse in cold or humid weather. Based on different scientific studies, between 70% and 100% suffer from depression, although this could be a result of suffering from the pain itself; 33% to 73% suffer from irritable bowel syndrome; 44% to 56% have severe headaches; 30% to 50% have white, cold hands (Raynaud's phenomenon); 24% suffer from anxiety; 18% have dry eyes and/or mouth (Sicca syndrome); 12% have Osteoarthritis; and 7% have Rheumatoid Arthritis.

Chaitow[8] also reports that other common conditions accompanying Fibromyalgia are allergies, almost constantly runny nose (chronic rhinitis), bruising easily, night cramps, restless leg syndrome, dizziness (sometimes because of medications taken for other symptoms), stopped breathing during sleep (apnea), dry eyes and mouth, teeth grinding (bruxism), extreme sensitivity to light (photophobia), premenstrual syndrome, digestive disturbances, viral infections, Lyme Arthritis Disease (resulting from a bacteria passed along by a tick), itchy skin — with or without rash — loss of hair, sensitive bladder, mouth ulcers, generalized muscular stiffness, 'foggy' brain (difficulty in concentrating and poor short-term memory), during reading wrong words come out, or the material is poorly understood (dyslexia), panic attacks, phobias, mood swings, irritability, and a feeling of hands and feet being swollen without evidence of fluid retention. There may also be a history of injury, major or minor, within the past year prior to start of the symptoms.

R. Paul St. Amand, M.D.,[4] Assistant Clinical Professor Medicine, Endocrinology-Harbor-UCLA, Marina del Rey, California, reports that "Today, Fibromyalgia is accepted as a distinct illness." In addition to the symptoms described above, he lists, nervousness; depression; impaired memory and concentration; headaches; blurring of vision; eye irritation; sensations of heat, flushing or actual sweating; sugar craving; nasal congestion; post-nasal drip; abnormal tastes (foul or metallic); transient ringing or other sounds; numbness and tingling anywhere but usually of hands and feet; gas and bloating; constipation alternated often with diarrhea; burning on urination; pungent urine; frequent bladder infections especially in women; vaginal irritation, discharge, pain and especially with intercourse and increased menstrual cramping; restless; leg cramps frequent; brittle nails; itching with or without various rashes, all subject to cyclic appearances, sometimes better, sometimes worse.

Most of the above symptoms also clearly fit those of Candidiasis, infestation by *Candida albicans* (and related organisms) which we presume will often accompany any of the rheumatoid diseases, including Fibromyalgia. (See *Arthritis: Osteoarthritis and Rheumatoid Disease Including Rheumatoid Arthritis*; *Conquering Yeast Infections*; *Dr. Crook Discusses Yeasts and How They Can Make You Sick*; *The Yeast Syndrome*, and "Candidiasis: Scourge of Arthritics," http://www.arthritistrust.org.)

According to St. Amand, "Many Fibromyalgics suffer primarily fatigue, emotional and cognitive defects and complain less of pain and other symptoms. This presentation is often labeled "chronic fatigue syndrome" and has been attributed to Ebstein-Barr or other viruses. It is progressively recognized as merely a facet of the same disease with symptoms predominantly at one end of a spectrum. To us, 'systemic candidiasis' and 'myofascial pain syndrome' are merely symptoms for Fibromyalgia."[4]

Dr. St. Amand says, "The most prevalent areas of pain are: shoulder muscles or tendons, neck, between shoulder blades, lower back often with sciatica. The knees, inner and outer elbow regions, wrists, hips and chest are equally frequent sources of discomfort. However, other sites are so often involved, pain should be expected from any skeletal muscle, tendon, ligament or fascia. Morning, flu-like, generalized stiffness is common. Previously injured or operative sites are often affected. . . . I believe that Fibromyalgia is the early phase of a complex disease leading to Osteoarthritis. Damage to cartilage and arthritic spurs do not appear overnight. Years of pain and often joint swelling occur before discernable X-ray changes."[4]

Symptom Confusions

According to Leon Chaitow, D.O.,[8] chronic fatigue syndrome and Fibromyalgia seem to start in the same way and to have the same symptoms, except that for the former, the fatigue element is most prominent, while for the latter, the muscle pain is the most prominent.

Others have debated as to whether or not Fibromyalgia and other forms of muscle, or myofascial, pain is the same. Literally dozens of different words have already been used to describe essentially the same physical conditions.

There is no evidence that Fibromyalgia is a disease of the muscles or a rheumatic syndrome.[11] Magnetic Resonance imaging is unable to depict any primary skeletal muscle abnormality, and there is no symptom of pain in those who are exercised and physically fit.[12]

Still others have used the name Fibrositis, meaning "inflammation of the muscles," where no inflammation can be found. By changing the name to Fibromyalgia syndrome, the implication of inflammation can be dropped, but even so, the cluster of symptoms as a unique disease entity remains not well defined.

Causation for Bursitis and Fibromyalgia

Bursitis may be caused by trauma, acute or chronic infection, inflammatory arthritis, Gout or Rheumatoid Arthritis.

Fibrositis pains can be brought on or intensified by trauma, exposure to dampness and cold, and by rheumatic problems. A virus or toxemia — the effect of absorption of bacterial toxins or products formed at a local source of infection — are felt to be causative sources.

Fibromyalgic pain is believed to be a self-maintained (neurophysiologic) disturbance where external stresses somehow interfere with sleep patterns resulting in increased pain perception. [There is deterioration of the non-rapid eye movement (REM) sleep]. The increased pain leads to additional stress and — altogether typical feedback characteristics — where one causative physiological disturbance produces the second

A hypothesis consistent with the idea that Fibromyalgic pain is a self-maintained disturbance has been put forth by Drs. Guy E. Abraham, M.D. and Jorge D. Flechas, M.D., M.P.H.[33]³ "Synthesis of proteins, fats and carbohydrates necessary for cellular integrity, normal activity and functions is dependent on adenosine triphosphate (ATP) availability which supplies the energy for their synthesis and actions." Synthesis in this ATP energy cycle requires the presence of oxygen, magnesium, inorganic phosphate and other substances. When these are present in optimum concentration, the integrity of the mitochondrial membrane wherein lies the ATP power unit and the capacity of the enzymatic system becomes enhanced. Without sufficient ingredients, the ATP energy cycle is inhibited.

Linda Simon, D.C. reports that "It has been found that the tender points of Fibromyalgia patients are sites of small lesions or tears (microlesions) in the muscle. These microlesions tense up or contract. Contracted fibers cause the muscle to shorten. Within the areas of contracted muscle, tiny blood vessels are compressed, greatly reducing the blood flow.

"Several things happen when blood flow is reduced to muscles. The muscle fibers become starved for oxygen (which is supplied by the blood cells) causing the surrounding muscle fibers to go into further spasm. The increased spasm prevents blood flow even further, creating a vicious cycle of spasm and loss of blood flow. Now more and more muscles are involved.

"At the areas of decreased blood flow, pain-producing chemicals (eg. bradykinins) are released. These chemicals are picked up by special nerve sites (nociceptors) in the muscles. According to Dr. Karl Hendriksson, 'abundant and continued pain provoking chemicals can lead to changes in the way the brain receives the pain information.' Normally most of the pain signals are blocked in the nervous system before they reach the brain. However, in the case of Fibromyalgia, Dr. Hendriksson has hypothesized that the constant release of pain-producing chemicals sensitizes the nerve sites (nociceptors) in the muscles, thus causing them to continually transmit pain signals."[41]

When there are no associated arthritic or hormonal conditions, this disturbance is called "Primary Fibromyalgia."

In Secondary Fibromyalgia, there is associated: rheumatic diseases such as Systemic Lupus Erythematosus, Rheumatoid Arthritis, Osteoarthritis, Fibromyalgic states of endocrine problems (endocrinopathies), rapid corticosteroid reduction (if having been on this drug), alcohol and narcotic withdrawal.

Although trigger points can also be identified with myofascial pain, pressure to these points will cause the pain to radiate to the entire area, which is not true with Fibromyalgic states.

Alan H. Pressman, D.C., Ph.D. reports that, "There is now a considerable body of evidence indicating that many of these . . . disease conditions are associated with a permeable gut, liver detoxification pathways and activation of the pain-producing inflammatory cascade."[10]

Peter Smrz, M.D. says: ". . . we also encounter bacterial infections which occur in conjunction with articular (joint) complaints. The most severe form here may be considered to be streptococcus-related rheumatism as it develops after scarlet fever or angina tonsillaris."[58]

Based on observations, R. Paul St. Amand, M.D. suspects that the primary defect in the production of Fibromyalgia lies with phosphate not calcium metabolism. "Calcium tablets taken with meals allowed lower dosages of [guaifenesin] medications. Calcium and magnesium bind phosphates from food, increase fecal excretion and thereby lessen absorption. Some patients have fingernail changes that suggest an abnormal calcium phosphate deposition at the root. Similar to concentric tree rings, they grow and eventually break or peel at the tip. Primarily phosphate — some calcium oxalate — increased in the urine as we initiated treatment in the few patients we tested. Our hypothesis is that an inherited, abnormal renal retention of phosphate and secondarily, calcium, leads to an intracellular excess of both. Cells and their power stations, the mitochondria, malfunction and produce inadequate ATP, the currency of energy. An energy deprivation syndrome develops and affects susceptible, widespread, bodily functions. We realize this is simplistic and the chemistry would be far more involved."[4]

Traditional Treatments

While conservative treatment may begin with non-steroidal anti-inflammatory drugs (NSAIDS), such as aspirin, and other over-the-counter "arthritis" remedies, traditional treatment for Fibromyalgia usually involves medication, a carefully designed exercise program, and sympathetic support. This combination of factors is said to "help" approximately 80% of the patients. It is only symptomatic treatment, at best.

Low doses of amitriptyline or cyclobenzaprine are prescribed to improve the sleeping pattern, causing drowsiness and later awakening with less fatigue and pain.

13

Swimming or rhythmic dancing is encouraged.

Although the patient will understand that Fibromyalgia is not a crippling or deforming disease, they must learn to deal with stress.

With the use of traditional treatments, and despite any of the above treatments, tender points will persist.

However, R. Paul St. Amand, M.D.[4] describes a "traditional" treatment that provides reversal of all the symptoms of Fibromyalgia under some rather strict rules.

The main substance used is guaifenesin, often combined with other ingredients for both over-the-counter and prescription medications. Guaifenesin by Dr. St. Amand is used without mixing with any other ingredients in the amount usually of 300 mg tablets twice a day for two weeks, which is an adequate dosage for about 20% of those afflicted. Six hundred milligram dosages are used for 50% more of the patients, and another 30% will need larger dosages. Once a proper dosage level is established for a given patient, treatment continues for two months, a time usually adequate to reverse at least one year of accumulated disease. "The longer the duration of illness, the longer the total clearing time."[4]

Of course, Dr. St. Amand also relies on a detailed medical history, examinations and so on as is customary.

In rare instances side effects may include nausea, heartburn, itching, or rash, but otherwise the treatment is safe and may be used at any age level.

Of significant importance for this treatment to be effective, is the total avoidance of salicylic acid which is often unknowingly used in skin ointments, herbs, aspirin and other pain relievers. St. Amand cautions that the patient should avoid such things as aloe, ginseng, menthol, mentholatum, almond oil, . . . castor and camphor oils, eyeliners, some lipsticks and underarm deodorants." This applies to sun screens, hair sprays, astringents, shaving creams, exfoliants, wart and callous removers, Peptobismol, some mouthwashes, and so on. "These offending substances will be absorbed and partially or totally block the effect of guaifenesin. No adverse reaction ensues but no benefit is attained."[4] Although all plants contain salicylates (or salicylic acid), the ban does not include foods, cooking herbs and spices, as the amount of salicylate contained is too small to effectively block guaifenesin. Non-steroidal inflammatory drugs that do not contain any salicylates are permitted.

After proper dosage has been determined the patient will develop an accelerated process of symptom reversal, having some good days and some bad days.

Clinical Symptoms for Bursitis

Acute Bursitis is characterized by pain, local tenderness, and limitation of motion. Swelling and redness is frequently present if the bursa is superficial.

Chronic Bursitis may follow prior attacks, or repeated trauma or foci of

14

infection. The bursal wall is thickened, with degeneration of the tissue surrounding the bone (endothelial lining). The bursa may eventually contain adhesions, threadlike processes from the synovial membrane (villi), calcium (calcareous) deposits and muscle atrophy.

Pain, swelling, tenderness, muscle weakness and limitation of motion vary.

Attacks may last from a few days to several weeks, with multiple recurrences.

Tendon or muscle tears must be ruled out, as well as inflammation of the bone marrow (osteomyelitis), tuberculosis, and inflammation of connective tissue or cells (cellulitis).

The elbow (olecranon bursa) and the knee (prepatellar bursa) are the most frequent sites of bursitis in children.

The knee (prepatellar bursa) is the most frequent site in adults.

Areas of abnormal stress, such as prominent bunions or amputation stumps, can acquire bursar sacs.

Subcutaneous bursitis associations or sources include trauma, bacterial infection, Gout, and Rheumatoid Arthritis. Such cases manifest as a cystic lump. When inflammation is severe or a bursae ruptures, diagnoses can be confused.

To differentiate between acute arthritis and Bursitis, the elbow, knee or limb is held in a semiflexion position, and passive extension or flexion is prevented because of pain, indicating acute arthritis.

For example: Holding the arm outward at a right angle to the body would be a half-open or half-closed position of the joint at the shoulder. Moving the arm from the leg to this half-open position would be painful for an inflamed bursae, whereas, continued raising of the arm, over the head, would not be painful with an inflamed bursae, but would be painful for one with acute arthritis. Similar, knee and limb positions would produce like results.

A bursal rupture will often show massive forearm and hand swelling (edema), suggesting inflammation of cartilage or cellular tissue (cellulitis) or vein clot (thrombosis).

The greater majority of cases of Bursitis due to infection (septic Bursitis) are due to *Staphylococcous aureus*.

Clear fluids with low white blood count (WBC) are common in Bursitis caused by infection and also in Gout. Routine analysis must include a uric acid crystal search by polarizing microscopy, Gram stain, and cultures.

Traditional Treatment for Bursitis

Subcutaneous Bursitis

Most traditional treatments for Bursitis are conservative, as most cases resolve spontaneously within three months if repetitive trauma is avoided by the patient. A conservative treatment normally involves non-steroidal anti-inflammatory drugs (NSAIDS), such as aspirin, and, although often prescribed,

15

over-the-counter "arthritis" remedies to inhibit pain.

Cases that do not respond are usually treated with a corticosteroid injection or even by surgery on the "offending" bursar sac.

Corticosteroids will often produce skin atrophy and infections due to repeated intra-bursae hyperdermic needles. When this occurs, a ten day course of antibiotics of one kind or another is prescribed, usually orally, but sometimes intravenously for patients with diabetes, or who suffer from immunosuppression, or suspected bacterial infections.

Deep Bursitis

While there are more than 100 deep bursae, only five of them seem to be of clinical importance: (1) beneath the outward extension of the spine of the scapula, forming the point of the shoulder (subacromion), creating shoulder pain; (2) at the neck of the femur (trochanteric), creating hip pain; (3) inside of the leg, below the knee (pes anserine); (4) back of the knee (gastrocnemius-semimembranosus), creating knee pain; and (5) behind the heel bone (retrocalcaneal), creating heel pain.

Traditional Treatment for Deep Bursitis

Usually corticosteroid injections at the sites of inflammation symptomatically dampen the pain and inflammation.

What's Wrong With Traditional Treatments?

Except for the treatment described by R. Paul St. Amand, using guaifenesin, traditional treatments address only the symptoms of the disease, not its source or cause.

Analgesics, and non-steroidal anti-inflammatory drugs, over time, destroy the lining of the stomach, and create other ill effects that sometimes can add additional burdens to an already diseased body.

Sherry A. Rogers, M.D.[30] writes that the use of non-steroidal anti-inflammatory drugs make Fibromyalgia worse once it has started. "These drugs cause widening between cells in the intestinal or gut lining. This is called intestinal hyperpermeability, or the leaky gut syndrome. These large spaces allow toxins, bacterial products, and foods that the body normally does not see to pass into the bloodstream. When it sees these new or foreign particles, it mounts an attack and starts making antibodies to them. Hence, food allergies, for example, can surface. . . . Furthermore, the bacterial toxins that leak through can damage the liver and reduce its ability to handle other chemicals in the environment."

Tricyclic antidepressants, according to Leon Chaitow, D.O., "increase the amount of serotonin in the central nervous system, increase the delta-wave stage of sleep and consistently improve the symptoms of Fibromyalgia, though not by acting as an antidepressant and not in all sufferers treated.

"Studies involving various forms of antidepressant medication tend to support the use of amitriptyline (25 to 50 mg daily), with pain scores, stiffness,

16

sleep and fatigue symptoms all improving on average, but by no means in all sufferers. . . . side effects of taking the antidepressant were measurable . . . drowsiness, confusion, seizure, agitation, nightmares, blurred vision, hallucinations, uneven heartbeat, grastrointestinal upsets, low blood pressure, constipation, urinary retention, impotence and dryness of the mouth all being observed or reported in various combinations."[8]

Corticosteroids have many well-known damaging side-effects, including the impairment of wound healing, increasing the risk of infection, and upsetting the delicate balance of the immunological system. Over time, ever-larger dosages are required to achieve the same level of symptomatic relief, and, in time, the body's ability to produce its own cortisone-like substances diminishes until one becomes absolutely dependent upon the drug for life itself. Many other bodily functions are also disturbed, or permanently damaged by long-term corticosteroid usage.

As reported by Leon Chaitow, D.O., "A study of the use of systemic corticosteroids (15 mg daily of prednisone) showed that there were no measurable improvements in those taking them . . . ."[8]

Chaitow, D.O. also reports that "When muscle relaxants were tested as treatment for Fibromyalgia sufferers, most were found to be useless. However, cyclobenzaprine (10 to 40 mg daily, given at night to prevent daytime drowsiness) was found to reduce pain levels and tender point count and improve sleep."[8]

As Deep Bursitis may be caused by various factors, including infection, Gout, Osteoarthritis, Synovitis, and so on, these injections may need to be repeated from time to time, unless the source of the problem is corrected.

Some diseases mimic Fibrositis or Bursitis, among which are three:

A chronic generalized inflammatory condition of the large arteries — principally in the temple and back of the head — polymyalgia rheumatica — may appear to be Fibrositis, but is actually a distinct rheumatoid disease causing severe pain, stiffness and disability.

Another soft tissue condition that results from inflammation of the arteries is giant cell arteritis. Often lumped together with polymyalgia rheumatica, it can cause severe musculo-skeletal aches and pains, and in some cases blindness as well.

A type of neuralgia sensed as a burning or acute pain radiating along a nerve and its branches is called causalgia or reflex sympathetic dystrophy, a disease that might occur after a trivial injury, causing severe disability to a limb.

**Alternative Treatments for Bursitis, Rheumatism,
Fibromyalgia, Fibromyositis, Fibrositis**

According to Robert C. Atkins, M.D., author of *Dr. Atkins' Health Revolution*, "Arthritis, which really is a term for a number of pathological conditions affecting the joints, is a perfect proving ground for therapy-testing. It has features in common with most conditions we have been treating. It is widespread, chronic, has elements of allergy, autoimmunity, microorganism, and free radical involvement; it is related to diet, nutrition, and environmental influences. It is a discomforting, disabling, discouraging, degenerative disease.

"Arthritis even has the politico-economic protection of its own special interest group, the Arthritis Foundation, more determined than any of its counterparts to insure its own continued existence by hammering home the Big Lie that all treatments which are non-pharmaceutical are quackery.

"For all these reasons, you would do well to understand that whatever works in treating arthritis would work for most illnesses."[17]

The Case of Maria Diamante

Fifty-five year old Maria Diamante, a victim of Rheumatoid Arthritis, was in great pain, with difficulty in walking, when she first entered Robert C. Atkins' office. She was five feet one inch tall and weighed 152 pounds and, according to Dr. Atkins, had that "overblown look that overtreated rheumatoid victims have."

Maria had had two operations (gallbladder and thyroid) some years earlier, and she'd begun to have Bursitis in her shoulders. Orthodox practitioners gave her the usual cortisone injections, and after these started she began to complain of arthritis pain in all of her joints. Of course, the usual was then prescribed of Indocin®, gold injections and Motrin®, all of which failed, and so surgery was next recommended.

Maria had a bilateral hip replacement, and after the passage of four more years, both knees were replaced. Maria was still in pain, and so, next, surgery was performed on both big toes and then her right wrist.

This "radical intervention" (as physicians title the surgery) did nothing whatsoever to halt the progress of Maria's arthritis, so again she was placed on pharmaceuticals.

By the time Maria Diamante came to see Dr. Atkins, she was on aspirin, Naprosyn®, prednisone and hydrochlorothiazide, this last a diuretic given for the purpose of offsetting the side effects of Naprosyn and prednisone.

Maria's sedimentation rate was high, which is a laboratory sign of chronic inflammation when taken together with other blood factors. She was anemic and her bone-related serum enzyme (alkaline phosphatase) level was high. Maria's glucose tolerance test went through violent swings, confirming hypoglycemia along with high insulin levels, implying that her carbohydrate metabolism was not functioning properly. Hair analysis also pointed to iron deficiency.

Dr. Atkins removed Maria from aspirin and hydrochlorothiazide immediately, and also instructed her to refrain from eating the nightshades: tomatoes, potatoes, paprika, eggplant, green pepper, and (smoking) tobacco. Otherwise she was placed on the Atkins Center's low-carbohydrate diet, which

18

also helped to eliminate foods that are known to affect large numbers of people.

The first month Maria was given supplements that included, among other items, superoxide dismutase (SOD) and panthothenic acid.

The Second month she was given intravenous vitamin C, B complex, B[6], folic acid, zinc, manganese, and magnesium. Orally, she was given bromelain, one teaspoon of vitamin C crystals 3 times daily, and niacin at bedtime.

The third month Maria received six vitamin drips, and by now felt stronger and was more active.

Dr. Atkins felt that her medications should be removed gradually to prevent withdrawal symptoms from Naprosyn and prednisone, and as this withdrawal took place, Maria's condition accelerated, until "her complaints were limited to some numbness and tingling in her joints," the pain being now gone.

In another month Maria's ankles and wrists were virtually pain free, the wrist that had not been operated upon being more mobile and painless. She'd lost twenty pounds, and on each visit to Dr. Atkins' office, her condition showed improvement. She told Dr. Atkins, "When I first came to you, I could hardly walk. Now I don't think about it, I just walk without pain. I can even lift and use my right arm. I really feel good. Last month I broke my shoulder, so I had to go to the hospital, and not one doctor could believe what he saw. I was seen as a miracle. They couldn't believe how well and free of pain I am."[17]

Maria kept up her visits to the Atkins Center, and five years from her first visit, her improvement continued, Dr. Atkins reported.

Acupressure

Michael Reed Gach, author of several books describing the proper use of acupressure, quotes Norman Shealy, M.D., a world-renowned pain specialist and director of the pain rehabilitation center in La Crosse, Wisconsin. Dr. Shealy "has found several acupressure points to be useful in treating pain and has incorporated them into his overall pain reduction program, which can be used for arthritis pain."[19]

The Case of Leslie

Michael Gach describes Leslie, a fifty-eight-year-old widow, who "was searching for a drug-free way to relieve the pain and swelling of the arthritis in her hands and toes, as well as a variety of allergies. She had lost feeling in her toes, and her doctor had said that she had very slight chance of regaining feeling in them.

"After three months of acupressure treatments every week, she was able to flex her toes back and forth, and move them at will without pain. Slowly, feeling came back into her toes." Gach says, "I will never forget how excited Leslie was to be able to wiggle her toes."[19]

According to Murray C. Sokoloff, M.D., "Easily reversible conditions such as Fibromyalgia, Fibrositis, and Myofascial syndrome may go into complete remission with the help of acupressure treatments. Acupressure offers relief with no risk and at the same time is inexpensive and easily integrated into one's life."[18]

Since many of the well-defined "tender" spots accompanying Fibrositis correspond to also well-defined Chinese acuncture points, one can easily locate these points simply by pressing the areas where the pain concentrates. Instead of massaging these extremely sensitive points, hold it firmly for a few minutes, gradually decreasing the pressure until you find a balance between pain and pleasure.

Myotherapy

For almost fifty years, Bonnie Pruden has been getting the kinks out of thousands of stiff muscles with a technique called myotherapy. Her technique applies pressure to Fibromyalgic tender points, which denies those points oxygen. The muscles relax thereby alleviating the pain at those points. Then, by re-educating affected muscles through gentle stretching exercises, the muscles stay relaxed and pain-free.

Bonnie Pruden doesn't claim to know why or how this process works, but work it does. She's "developed very specific range-of-movement exercises — corrective exercises — that help retrain specific muscles.

"For a qiuck fix for back pain, for example, pressure is applied to a tender knot located in the back-pocket region. This is followed by simple and gentle leg stretches while the client lies on her side. These stretches are followed by pelvic tilts and sphincter-tightening/relaxing exercises. Focusing on the pelvic girdle area," Pruden explains, "also helps relieve incontinence, poor urine flow, and spastic vaginal muscles.

"In addition to myotherapy, I've developed a mini-minute daily exercise program that can be performed in bed, in the shower, or at work. The idea is to get you to remain active and permanently fix sore muscles. You must move often throughout the day.

"The retraining exercises and emphasis on daily movement are the major differences between my method and other trigger point therapies. With acupressure or shiatsu, for example, you can relieve the spasm and pain, but without teaching better muscle habits, the spasm may return."

Acupuncture

Reported by Leon Chaitow, D.O., in treating Fibromyalgia with acupuncture, Dr. P. Baldry feels it is necessary to repeat the treatment every two to three weeks for months or even years.

M. Penny Levin, Ph.D., a health psychologist in the Philadelphia area, who also practices in a holistic context, wrote via internet that "My interest in acupuncture began with my own experience. I developed a serious inflammatory arthritis following the birth of my children. It was frighteningly unresponsive to traditional Western medicine.

"After several years of struggling, my husband's chiropractor, who was learning acupuncture at the time, offered to attempt to treat this condition. Within just a few months, I was 20 pounds lighter, vastly more energetic, and nearly off of all medication.

"Over the past several years, both my practice and my personal health care have shifted steadily in the direction of alternative medicine."[21]

In one study, 70 patients were divided into two groups, one half of whom received acupuncture treatment, and the other half a sham procedure. The treated group showed significant improvement, and the control (non-treated) group showed none.[31]

Double-blind scientific studies performed by a Swiss research team in Geneva found that only the real acupuncture treatments — as opposed to the non-acupuncture points treated as a placebo — resulted in improvement by those suffering from Fibromyalgia. After the treatment, the group receiving the real acupuncture required more pressure on tender points to produce pain, and the amount of painkilling medicine required was less by half, the length of time of morning stiffness was reduced by a small amount. However, about 25% of those treated with acupuncture did not improve.[8]

Allergies and Chemical Sensitivities

Reported by Leon Chaitow, D.O.,[8] people with allergies and chemical sensitivities are more likely to suffer from Fibromyalgia than those who do not have allergies. "In a study at East Carolina University School of Medicine in 1992, involving approximately 50 people with hay fever or perennial allergic rhinitis (runny nose), it was found that around half those tested fitted the criteria for Fibromyalgia set by the American College of Rheumatology.... As about 5% of the general population have Fibromyalgia, that 49% of sufferers in the study had allergy points to there being a close link between these two conditions.... the foods that most commonly cause problems for many people with Fibromyalgia or chronic fatigue syndrome ... are wheat and dairy products, sugar, caffeine, aspartame, alcohol and chocolate."[8]

Regarding chemical sensitivities, "according to Professor Gunnar Hauser, M.D., of UCLA, 'Toxic exposure doesn't always occur in factories. There are many chemicals in our everyday environment (as well as those acquired from medical and social drug usage) that can lead to serious health problems, including household cleaners, new carpets, perfumes and certain types of paints'.

"All the symptoms associated with Fibromyalgia and chronic fatigue syndrome ... can result from such exposure."

Warren Levin, M.D. of New York City described Hazel Nelson as a woman deeply disturbed over her back pain. "I didn't even try to treat her back pain," Dr. Levin said, "but tested her for food allergies. When we discovered that she was allergic to wheat, and she refrained from eating it, her back pain went away by itself."[22]

Anti-Microorganism Therapy

As there seems to be a strong correlation between many forms of arthritis and genetic or developed sensitivity to the toxins or dead protein products of various microorganisms, broad spectrum anti-microorganism drugs are highly recommended, at least as a trial or preliminary treatment program. (See *Arthritis: Osteoarthritis and Rheumatoid Disease Including Rheumatoid Arthritis*; "The Roger Wyburn-Mason, M.D., Ph.D. Treatment for Rheumatoid Disease," and "Thomas McPherson Brown, M.D. Treatment of Rheumatoid Disease," http://www.arthritistrust.org. The arthritis book is available on Amazon.com.)

Aroma Therapy

Anti-inflammatory effects can be obtained from odors that stimulate, such as thyme, cinnamon and cloves, according to studies by Dr. Hildebret Wagner, Chair of the Institute of Pharmaceutical Biology at Ludwig Maximilian University in Munich, Germany. "Dr. Wagner suggests that the irritation caused by these oils stimulates the adrenal glands and triggers release of anti-inflammatory corticoid substances, the body's natural cortisone-like material."[4]

Dr. Schnaubelt reports that everlast (*Helichrysum italicum*) and eucalyptus (*Eucalyptus radiata*) relieve arthritis pains within moments of application[4]

Aroma therapy principally supplements, or complements, other treatments for arthritis. Additional oils that benefit other arthritic treatments, according to Roberta Wilson, author of *Aromatherapy for Vibrant Health & Beauty*, include: basil, benzoin, black pepper, cedarwood, chamomile, coriander, elemi, fennel, ginger, helichrysum, juniper, lemon, marjoram, myrrh, pine, rosemary, and vetiver. "These oils can ease pain and discomfort, reduce swelling, and relieve sore muscles," according to Roberta Wilson.[7]

Wilson describes three useful recipes for the arthritic: (1) Arthritis Bath Blend, (2) Arthritis Massage Blend, (3) Deep Relief Arthritis Oil.

The Arthritis Bath Blend consists of oils: 3 drops lemon, 2 drops coriander, 2 drops helichrysum and 2 drops marjoram. The patient drops these oils into a bathtub filled with warm water, gently dispersing them. Then, a leisurely soak is enjoyed for twenty to thirty minutes.

Used in the Arthritis Massage Blend, are oils: 1-1/2 ounces carrier, 1/2 ounce flaxseed, 6 drops chamomile, 4 drops marjoram, 3 drops coriander, 3 drops rosemary, 2 drops benzoin resin, 1 drop black pepper, and 1 drop ginger. The carrier oil poured into a clean container is added to the other oils, and gently turned upside down several times, or rolled between hands to blend the mixture. This mixture is massaged over joints and muscles as necessary.

Deep Relief Arthritis Oil consists of oils: 1-1/2 ounces carrier, 1/2 ounce flaxseed, 4 drops chamomile, 4 drops helichrysum, 4 drops lemon, 3 drops fennel, 3 drops juniper, 3 drops marjoram, and 2 drops ginger. After the flax-seed and carrier oil are mixed together, the essential oils are blended. The mixture is then applied to joints and muscles as needed.

Wilson also advises that the arthritic can "Soak Arthritis Bath Blend daily to relive pain and discomfort. Apply Arthritis Massage Blend over your entire body for detoxifying and pain-relieving effect. Massage Deep Relief Arthritis Oil into your joints and muscles as often as necessary to relieve pain and reduce swelling."[7]

Bee Sting Therapy

The International Apitherapy Study begun in 1983, has gathered follow-up data on more than 12,000 bee stung patients. It may take up to 1-4 stings to reduce the pain of Bursitis.[50]

B6 Supplementation

The Case of Joseph G. Hattersley

Joseph G. Hattersley, medical reporter and writer, says, "I cured my own bursities in both shoulders 25 years ago with vitamin B6. And a Toastmasters friend, a rather large person, was out of work about 6 weeks ago, had $100 left in the bank, and was newly crippled with a painful knee. I told him if it was Bursitis, B6 would help — and handed him a bottle of the tablets. Now he takes 500 mg a day (with B-complex) and his pain is entirely gone. He doesn't run and jump much because of his size, but he sure does walk, and enjoys it."[44]

Research of John Marion Ellis, M.D.

John Marion Ellis, M.D., over a period of seven years of research with Dr. Karl Folkers and associates at the University of Texas, Austin, Texas, made many videotapes of before and after conditions of patients who, through the elimination of vitamin B6 deficiency, became well or, at least, vastly improved.

Dr. Folkers and other scientists were able to demonstrate that a particular enzyme — erthrocyte glutamic oxaloacetic transanimase (EGOT) — as measured in the blood, would confirm deficiency of vitamin B6[5]

Their studies were able to link decreasing measures of the above enzyme with age — the highest values found in the newly born, the lowest, in those with age and disease. Furthermore, they were able to demonstrate that it took seventy days to get the enzyme up to speed, which is the approximate time for most patients to show improvement using 100 to 150 mg of pyridoxine daily.

Measured values of the blood content of erthrocyte glutamic oxaloacetic transanimase (EGOT) enzyme were tabulated as follows:

0.12-0.20 (Irreversible Crippling)
0.20-0.30 (Pathological)
0.30-0.35 (Marginal)
0.35-0.40 (Biochemically Questionable)

Newly born infants will have an enzyme measure of 0.71, and those who take 50-100 mgs of B6 daily register at 0.69.

Most of the American population probably lays between 0.20 and 0.40, Dr. Ellis believed, indicating that a nationwide deficiency existed.[5]

<u>Signs and Symptoms of Vitamin B6 Deficiency</u>

As Rheumatoid Disease seems to be a grab-bag of virtually all auto-immune and collagen tissue diseases, Bursitis — also a Rheumatoid Disease — seems to be its equivalent in "soft-tissue," auto-immune/collagen tissue diseases.

Dr. Ellis and associates were able to show that the signs and symptoms of vitamin B6 deficiency may include the following:

1. Numbness and tingling of the hands (paresthesia);
2. Impaired finger sensations;
3. Limitations on ability to flex joints;
4. Swelling of hands that improves and worsens, or fluctuates;
5. Morning stiffness of finger joints;
6. Pain in the hands;
7. Coordination impairment of finger joints;
8. Weakness of pinch pressure between thumb and index finger;
9. Dropping of objects;
10. Tenderness over the Carpal Tunnel with neurological signs (Tinel and Phalen);
11. Painful shoulders;
12. Painful movement of thumb at knuckle (metacarpophalangeal joint);
13. Painful elbows;
14. "Sleep paralysis."

The above symptoms derive from the following list of conditions, all of which have been shown to respond to vitamin B6 therapy:

1. Carpal Tunnel Syndrome (Idiopathic);
2. Chronic noninflammatory Tenosynovitis (acute, sub-acute and chronic);
3. Chronic noninflammatory Tendinitis (acute, sub-acute and chronic);
4. Synovitis of thumb tendons (De Quervain's Disease);
5. Diabetic neuropathy as related to Carpal Tunnel Syndrome;
6. Synovitis situated around several joints (periarticular);
7. Shoulder-hand syndrome;
8. Pre-menstrual swelling (edema);
9. Menopausal arthritis;
10. Swelling of hands and feet (edema) of pregnancy;
11. Effects of bacterial toxins (toxemia) of pregnancy;
12. Proliferation beneath arterial endothelium (arterial subendothelial proliferation);
13. Thickening, degeneration and inflammation of arteries (arteriosclero-

sis).

The Case of Nurse Angeline Johnson

Nurse Angeline Johnson reported to Dr. Ellis that she had swelling in her face, feet and fingers, as well as soreness in her finger joints, but that after a few hours of activity during the day, the swelling would subside. These, she reported, seemed to coincide with her menstrual cycle.

Dr. Ellis prescribed 50 milligrams of vitamin B6 for five days. After two days, Angeline's hands had improved, and on the third day, she was able to wear her rings again, use the typewriter, and she slept much better.

For twelve months thereafter Nurse Johnson took one 50-milligram tablet daily of vitamin B6 and suffered no pain in her hands, and had no pre-menstrual swelling. When Dr. Ellis asked her to go without the vitamin B6, she found the pain and swelling returned. It disappeared again by returning to her former supplementation of vitamin B6[5]

Although this approach obviously was right for Nurse Johnson, there can be other hormonal factors that must be attended to, Dr. Ellis cautions.

The Cases of Carrie Summons and Martha Robinson

Carrie Summons and Martha Robinson, both nearing menopause, were "troubled with bright-red, distinctly circumscribed nodes on the finger joints, one of the frequent symptoms of menopausal arthritis, known as Herberden's nodes," named after William Herberden who first recorded the phenomena in the 18th Century.

After eight weeks of therapy, using vitamin B6, the Herberden nodes subsided.[5]

The Case of Mattye Stuert

African-American Mattye Stuert had poor neuro-muscular coordination of hand and finger, and would easily drop dishes and other objects. She also was unable to write to her husband who was in the service, because her hand would "go to sleep." She experienced pain in her right hand.

Dr. Ellis injected her with pyridoxine hydrochloride, 50 milligrams, daily, every other day. After two weeks, her grasp was improved so that she could hold objects in her right hand without dropping them, and the "pins and needles," in her hands and arms had disappeared, and her arm no longer went to sleep, so that now she was able to write to her husband.[5]

Shoulder-hand Syndrome

According to Dr. Ellis, a form of arthritis known as "the shoulder-hand syndrome," characterized by swelling of the fingers and hands, and painful movement of the elbows and shoulders, often accompanies an acute myocardial infarction, or during the convalescence after such an attack. Dr. Ellis wrote, that "the age of a patient and the length of time he has been suffering has a great bearing upon his response to B6 therapy, but in every case of the 'shoulder-hand syndrome' I have treated with pyridoxine, there has been some improvment."[5]

Dr. Ellis writes, "You will notice that nowhere in the above list [The Signs and Symptoms of B6 Deficiency] is the word 'arthritis' mentioned, except in relation to menopausal arthritis, which is a specific complaint. . . . the majority of people believe they are suffering from arthritis, when in fact, it is more often than not, some other complaint. In fact, as a result of my research, I firmly believe that 90% of what is called arthritis . . . is, in reality, a biochemical change in synovium of tendons and joints, particularly in the fingers, thumbs, elbows, shoulders, knees and hips. With these changes in synovium, a person experiences swelling, pain and stiffness of the joints, symptoms that most men and women as well as doctors call 'arthritis.' . . . as Karl Fokers and I have proved, these conditions respond favorably to adequate amounts of pyridoxine, given over a period of 90 days. Many of my patients experienced relief in only a matter of weeks, but in the majority of cases, it does take about six weeks for the symptoms to start disappearing, and twelve weeks for a definitive response. In cases of severe stiffness, there will be gradual improvement up to a year."[6]

The Case of Billy Joe McGill

Billy Joe McGill, great-grandson of a former slave from Mississippi who had been sent to Texas as a wedding gift, was a concrete finisher. He was having difficulty doing his twelve hours daily professional chores.

Billy Joe was placed in a double-blind study, having a power of pinch that was a mere 8.5 pounds.

After the test was over, and the study unblinded, Billy Joe McGill was found to have taken 100 mg of vitamin B6 daily, while his power of pinch had advanced to 22.6 pounds in his right hand and 24 pounds in his left hand.[5]

Pyridoxal 5-Phosphate

Since the early days of Dr. Ellis' research, many physicians have learned to prefer the use of pyridoxal 5-phosphate, a metabolite of pyridoxine, to avoid possible adverse effects of over-dosage of the pyridoxine.

Soft Tissue Arthritis is Caused by Proven B6 Deficiency

Dr. Ellis further states that his view, that most of the 'arthritis' in the world today is a deficiency in vitamin B6, is substantiated by long years of research, proven in laboratory experiments, evidenced from before and after videotapes, and proven under stringent double-blind conditions "in conjunction with some of the top medical and scientific authorities in the country."[5]

B12 and Copper Supplementation

Richard A. Kunin, M.D., of San Francisco, California writes, "I've seen cases of Bursitis respond to B12 therapy, probably because the vitamin promotes blood cell development, hematopoiesis (the production and development of blood cells, usually in bone marrow), which draws iron out of the tissues in order to bind it to the porphyrin (a respiratory pigment) of hemoglo-

26

bin instead.

"In the tissues free iron is a potent source of free radicals (chemically active substances), which cause inflammation and aggravate arthritis. Locked in the hemoglobin, the iron is perfectly safe; but in order to get there it must traverse the liver and accept an electron, i.e., be electronically reduced by a protein, ceruloplasmin (a glycoprotein, blue in color, to which the majority of the copper in blood is attached).

"Ceruloplasmin, however, is dependent on copper for its structure, and it is copper which signals the liver to manufacture the ceruloplasmin. Since copper is in short supply in the diet of about 3 out of 4 Americans, combined iron-copper deficiency is common. Many is the case of iron deficiency anemia that responds only when copper is supplied as well as iron.

"Low iron status causes tired bones as well as tired blood and tired people. Iron is essential for synthesis of collagen. Often the first symptom of iron deficiency is low back pain. that's where the maximum load occurs, upwards of 750 pounds leverage force is not unusual. If the collagen repair is slow, due to multiplicity of deficiencies, strain can lead to inflammation."[23]

One must be very careful, however, not to conclude that iron deficiency is a problem without proper laboratory measures as well as knowledgeable physician supervision. Adeena Robinson, *Iron: A Double Edged Sword*, suffering from "undiagnosable" symptoms eventually learned that she was a victim of iron overload. Iron overload, through arbitrary supplementations or however obtained, can cause liver dysfunction, enhance growth of cancer, supports infectious diseases, is a culprit in arthritis, especially among those whose Rheumatoid Factor (RF) is negative, is correlated with increased risk of heart disease and diabetes, can damage the pancreas, affect endocrine system, sexual functioning, and neurological disorders, and shows up in measures of metabolism in multiple sclerosis and cystic fibrosis.

Coupled with proper laboratory tests as described in *Iron: A Double Edged Sword*, specific signs and symptoms may lead the knowledgeable physician to conclude that iron overload is a factor in otherwise confusing disease symptoms, and blood letting (blood donations) or a chelating agent (desferrioxamine) may be recommended. (Caution: See a knowledgeable physician.)

Candidiasis

Dr. Carol Jessop reported that nearly 90% of her patients with Fibromyalgia, whether men or women, had yeast infections, probably because of their recurrent use of antibiotics for sinus, acne, prostate, urinary tract and chest infection problems.[8]

As there is a decided connection between candidiasis, food allergies, chemical sensitivities, and every form of arthritis, detoxifying the body by every safe, possible means is clearly in order for those suffering from Fibromyalgia. (See

27

Arthritis: Osteoarthritis and Rheumatoid Disease Including Rheumatoid Arthritis; *Conquering Yeast Infections*; *Dr. Crook Discusses Yeasts and How They Can Make You Sick*; *The Yeast Syndrome*, and "Candidiasis: Scourge of Arthritics," http://www.arthritistrust.org.)

Chiropractic

Chiropractic adjustments have been successful in treating various disturbances of the body, including Bursitis,[4] but may not consist solely of adjustments. Progressive doctors of chiropractic are frequently involved with nutrition and metabolic problems.

A case of mixed arthritis and Rheumatism is reported by Paul A. Goldberg, M.P.H., D.C.,[51] graduate of Bowling Green State University, Life College, and the University of Texas Medical Center Graduate School of Public Health. Dr. Goldberg, with degrees in preventive medicine, nutrition and chiropractic, was Professor of Clinical Nutrition, Gastroenterology and Rheumatology at Life College, Marietta, Georgia, and practices at The Goldberg Clinic in Marietta, Georgia.

The Case of Vickie Garrett

Vickie Garrett, 52-years-of-age, had a generalized chronic fatigue coupled with a 7 year history of joint/muscle pain and indigestion which was getting worse. She'd been taking "Herbal Formula" recommended by a "herbalist." When Vickie had begun using it 6 months earlier there'd been dramatic reduction in discomfort, but each week she had to increase the amount of the compound to receive the same effect, and her symptoms worsened.

Laboratory studies included blood chemistry, sedimentation rate (elevated), and amino acid profile (low). Her diet was analyzed and found inadequate.

Vickie was placed on an individualized program to improve her digestive function and to restore nutrient competency. She was also urged to rest and to discontinue the use of the herbal formula. Withdrawal from the herbal formula exacerbated her symptoms, and on further investigation the herbs were found to contain steroid compounds.

Vickie was asked to eliminate refined foods, increase essential nutrients, and to avoid food allergens. Her gut was rested with a week long liquid diet. Essential fatty acids and an amino acid mixture was recommended based on her blood analysis.

Following withdrawal symptoms that resulted from discontinuing the Herbal Formula, Vickie experienced gradual improvement in symptoms and an increase in energy. As her digestion improved, so did her joint and muscle pain. Sedimentation rate returned to normal, as did the amino acid levels.

Follow-up in 2 years found the patient reporting 90% improvement in overall health.

Dr. Goldberg says that "This patient exemplified the importance of good digestion. With digestion improved, amino acids, fatty acids, minerals and other nutrients became available to tissues for repair while inflammatory compounds entering the bloodstream reduced."

The Case of Joy Climer

Thirty-three-year-old Joy Climer came to Dr. Goldberg with a mixture of Fibromyositis and "mixed" arthritis. She experienced swelling and pain in ankles, shoulders and stiffness in other joints and muscles. There was ankle swelling and pain to the point that she found herself unable to walk. She also had indigestion with bloating and stomach pains.

Joy was found to have increased intestinal permeability, numerous food allergies and an elevated sedimentation rate.

A program was given to reduce gut permeability, eliminate allergens and improve digestion. A period of detoxification was followed by a special dietary program with nutrient supplements to assist in gut wall repair.

In 2 months the joint and muscle pain disapeared, her energy level increased, and her sedimentation rate returned to normal, as did gut permeability.

Control of Fibromyalgia Syndrome

Dr. Christiane Northrup[34] writes that "Biopsies of muscles of the tender points of Fibromyalgia patients have shown evidence of tissue damage resulting from decreased oxygenation of the tissue." Women, who suffer more from Fibromyalgia Syndrome than do men, by 9 to 1, "often have decreased blood supply to their muscles because of chronic muscular tension," which, Dr. Northrup feels, is caused by muscular tension caused by suppressed emotion stemming from thoughts, feelings and beliefs, probably related to job-created stress, family problems, or latent childhood memories.

Dr. Northrup sets out 6 major guidelines for control of Fibromyalgia, as follows:

1. Don't be afraid to exercise. Slowing down because your body signals to do so is not a good idea. No matter how you feel, continue moving every day, and over time your body will be able to tolerate moderate exercise as your muscles become conditioned and the pain decreases.

2. Get plenty of rest and relaxation. Try for 8 to 10 hours of sleep each night, and go to bed and arise at the same time each day, even on weekends. "A definite schedule helps train your body to rest deeply and fully when you are in bed. (Remember, the key is quality sleep, not necessarily quantity.)"

3. Meditate. Meditation helps to balance neurotransmitter hormones. "Just 15 minutes per day will do wonders for all aspects of your life — not just relieving your Fibromyalgia Syndrome."

4. Eat a diet that optimizes the prostaglandin hormone balance in your cells. An unbalanced intake of the wrong kind of prostaglandin hormones, usually derived from the wrong kind of fatty acids, causes tissue inflammation resulting in muscle pain. The right kind of fatty acids, such as derives from

the Omega-3 and Omega-6 sources, — alpha linolenic acid, eicosapentaenoic acid, docosahexaenoic acid, and gamma linolenic acid (from flax oil, walnuts and beans, whole grains, chestnuts, soybeans, cold water non-farmed ocean fish, Evening Primrose seeds, Black Currant seeds and Borage seeds, for example) — have an opposite effect, by helping to dampen inflammation as well as other benefits.

"A diet that is low in refined carbohydrates, low in fat, and moderate in protein keeps prostaglandin hormone tissue levels well balanced. Also, eat no more than 500 calories in one sitting — a huge meal taxes your system and disrupts your natural rhythms. Include a bit of protein and fat at each meal or snack. This keeps prostaglandin levels in balance by keeping insulin levels steady."

5. Increase serotonin levels in your blood. Dr. Northrup explains that researchers have been able to produce Fibromyalgia-like symptoms by decreasing the neurotransmitter serotonin. The reason why doctors give small amounts of antidepressants for Fibromyalgia is because these drugs artifically increase serotonin.

"Anything that makes you happy and enthusiastic tends to increase your serotonin levels. . . . You can also boost your serotonin with blue-green algae."

Blue-green algae consists of whole algae, rich in amino acids, chlorophyll, enzymes, nucleic acids, essential fatty acids, vitamins, naturally chelated minerals, including trace minerals, and natural sugars. Some brands have a higher overall amino acid content than others, including the raw materials for building neuropeptides, and some brands retain live enzymes.[38]

Dr.Northrup feels that it is important to take these supplements "in a progressive and regular pattern," and she offers the following regimen:

Week One: Take two digestive enzyme capsules with blue-green algae just before breakfast and lunch. Also, take two acidophilus capsules with algae each morning 30 minutes before eating. ("Friendly Bacteria -- Lactobacillus acidophilus & Bifido bacterium," http://www.arthritistrust.org.)

Week Two: Add blue-green algae at breakfast each day.

Week Three: Stay with the enzymes and acidophilus, but begin increasing your algae intake to 2-5 capsules three times per day with meals.

Week Four: Continue to experiment with the amount of algae you need. Some people get very good results with just a little, while others require a heftier intake.

6. Take supplements. Dr. Northrup states that "Magnesium, malic acid, manganese, and the B vitamins have all been shown to decrease pain in Fibromyalgia Syndrome patients. Magnesium and malic acid help the body synthesize energy and strengthen cell membranes, thus preventing microtrauma to the muscles. They also help with aluminum detoxification (excess aluminum

may be implicated in Fibromyalgia Syndrome, but results are inconclusive as of yet).

"Take a total of 300-600 mg of magnesium daily, either in your multivitamin/mineral supplement or separately.

"For malic acid, start with 1,200 mg per day in divided doses with meals. You can gradually increase to 2,400 mg per day if you experience no pain relief within the first two weeks.

"The B vitamins support cell wall healing and most other metabolic functions": 100 mg each of the B's.

"Manganese is a necessary co-factor in the production of neurotransmitters": 10-20 mg of manganese.

Dr. Northrup says that she routinely has good results in 3 to 6 weeks when she places her Fibromyalgia patients on the above regimen.[34]

Diet and Nutritional Supplements
Modified Cave Man Diet

(Consistent with Dr. Christiane Northrup's regimen, consider use of the diet described in *Arthritis: Osteoarthritis and Rheumatoid Disease Including Rheumatoid Arthritis,* "and/or "Lonsdale Diet: Why I Left Orthodox Medicine," i http://www.arthritistrust.org). Most healthy diets remind us that fresh fruits, vegetables, whole grains, nuts and cold-water fish is closer to our caveman ancestors' diets, and also the diet that followed man's evolution. Modify this diet according to your doctor's instructions. Eat foods high in magnesium: dark leafy greens, and green and yellow vegetables.[4]

Zoltan Rona, M.D., M.Sc.[35] was asked by a 33-year-old mother of three children for advice. She explained that she was on Tylenol® 3 (with codeine), Demerol®, Diauldid®, Prozac®, Immovane®, Diazepam®, and Sinequain®. She wanted to know if she could do anything healthier.

Dr. Rona's reply was, "The number and combination of drugs you are taking is alarming. Your first order of business should be to wean off the drugs with the help of a drug detoxification centre. Once this is accomplished look into natural approaches to treatment. (See "Allergies and Biodetoxification for the Arthritic," http://www.arthritistrust.org.)

"Foods that should be reduced are refined carbohydrates (sugar and white flour products) and animal fats (especially those found in red meats)."

Dr. Rona also advised taking the correct kind of essential fatty acids, similar to advice already described above by Dr. Christiane Northrup and other physicians.

Dr. Rona added that the Fibromyalgia sufferer should "Avoid foods known to interfere with mineral absorption such as bran, coffee and tea."

Supplemental "minerals that may be useful include iron, zinc, copper, manganese, calcium, magnesium, silicon, boron and selenium.

"Vitamins such as A, B-complex, C, beta-carotene, bioflavonoids and E can be supplemented in higher than RDA doses because they are antioxidants."

Dr. Rona also reports the beneficial use of alfalfa, calendula, intramuscular injections of B12, magnesium sulphate, and the use of natural progesterone, liothyronine (thyroid replacement T3), the hormone replacement dehydroepiandrosterone (DHEA), the amino acid typtophan and electroacupuncture.[35] (See "Thyroid Hormone Therapy: Cutting the Gordian Knot," http://www.arthritistrust.org.)

Potassium-Magnesium Aspartate

Alan R. Gaby, M.D. recommends potassium-magnesium aspartate for tired people, i.e., those with chronic fatigue syndrome, a condition that has many symptoms in common with Fibromyalgia. Dr. Gaby reports "that potassium-magnesium aspartate is frequently an effective treatment for fatigue. This compound is said to be helpful regardless of the cause of the fatigue."[9]

Nutritionist Nan Kathryn Fuchs, Ph.D.[15] reports that when large amounts of calcium are taken as supplements, or through dietary regimens, calcium is increased in the blood, which stimulates the secretion of a hormone called calcitonin. The parathyroid hormone is also suppressed, and these two hormones regulate the levels of calcium found in bones, tissues and teeth, and have a direct relationship to the degree of Osteoporosis and Osteoarthritis. Also, parathyroid hormone takes calcium out of bones and deposits it in soft tissues while calcitonin is depositing calcium in bones.

The correct balance resulting from moving calcium about in the body is obtained only when there is sufficient magnesium, because magnesium suppresses the parathyroid hormone and stimulates calcitonin. "This chemical action helps prevent Osteoarthritis and Osteoporosis," Dr. Fuchs says. "A magnesium deficiency, however, will prevent this chemical action. And more calcium is not the solution, because while magnesium helps the body absorb and utilize calcium, excessive calcium prevents the absorption of magnesium. Taking more calcium without adequate magnesium — and what is adequate for one woman may be insufficient for another — may either create calcium malabsorption or a magnesium deficiency."[15] (See "Prevention and Treatment of Osteoarthritis,"Treatment and Prevention of Osteoporosis," and "Magnesium Chloride HexahydrateTherapy," http://www.arthritistrust.org.)

In a study reported by Dr. Fuchs, "Volunteers on a low magnesium diet were given both calcium and vitamin D supplements. All subjects were magnesium-deficient, and all but one became deficient in calcium as well, in spite of the fact that calcium had also been added to their diet. When they were given intravenous calcium infusions, the level of calcium in their blood rose for the duration of the intravenous feedings. When intravenous calcium was stopped, blood levels of calcium dropped again. However, when they were given magnesium, their magnesium levels rose rapidly and stabilized, and their

32

calcium levels also rose within a few days, even though they had not been given any additional calcium."[15]

Fibromyalgia sufferer, David Squires, says that "Malic acid is one of the ingredients that aids the body in the adenosene triphosphate (ATP) process (the cell's energy cycle). Malic acid occurs naturally in fruits and vegetables and normally is produced in the body while metabolizing sugars to make adenosene triphosphate (ATP). However, one published study has shown that this process is abnormal in Fibromyalgia and chronic immune dysfunction syndrome (CFIDS), and that sufficient malic acid may not be formed. In addition, four studies have indicated that adenosene triphosphate (ATP) is lower than normal in these syndromes. The adenosene triphosphate (ATP) process is magnesium dependent."[24] To Your Health, Inc., founded by David Squires and his family, therefore recommends magnesium glycinate, which, he says, "is easy to digest and readily absorbed into the blood stream." Other ingredients included in their Fibro-Care ^{TM} are manganese which complements the blend by stimulating the production of thyroxin, a hormone that influences the ceullar metabolic rate; two B vitamins, thiamine B1 and pyridoxine B6 which work closely with magnesium in the energy production process. Deficiency in thiamine metabolism, Squires reports, "has been found by one group of investigators to be abnormal." (See David Squires. "Fibromyalgia — David's Story," *A Resource Catalog*, To Your Health, Inc., 11809 Nightingale Circle, Fountain Hills, Arizona 85268.)

Magnesium and Malic Acid

Guy E. Abraham, M.D. and Jorge D. Flechas, M.D., M.PH.[33] in an open clinical setting gave 15 patients ages 32-60 oral preparations of Super Malic® from Optimax Corporation, Torrance, CA, containing 50 mg of magnesium hydroxide and 200 mg of malic acid per tablet. A total daily dosage of 300-600 mg of magnesium and 1200-1400 of malic acid was administered.

Assessed by the use of a Tender Point Index (TPI), an American College of Rheumatology 1990 criteria, all patients reported significant improvement within 48 hours of starting the treatment.

After 6 weeks, 6 patients were switched to a placebo tablet for 2 weeks. Recurrence of Fibromyalgia occurred within 48 hours in all patients who, unknowingly, were on the placebos.

Magnesium Chloride Hexahydrate Therapy

According to Raul Vergini, M.D..[14] Predappio, Italy, back in 1915, a French surgeon, Prof. Pierre Delbet, M.D., was looking for a solution to cleanse wounds, because he had found out that the traditional antiseptic solutions actually mortified tissues and facilitated the infection instead of preventing it.

He tested several mineral solutions and discovered that a magnesium chloride solution was not only harmless for tissues, but it had also a great effect

33

over leucocytic (blood cell) activity and phagocytosis; so it was perfect for external wounds treatment. Phagocytosis is the engulfing and perhaps the destroying of bacteria and other foreign bodies.

Dr. Delbet performed a lot of "in vitro" [in test tube] and "in vivo" [in life] experiments with this solution and he became aware that it was good not only for external applications, but it was also a powerful immuno-stimulant if taken by injections or even by mouth. He called this effect "cytophilaxis." In some "in vivo" experiments it was able to increase phagocytosis rate up to 300%.

Dr. Delbet serendipitously discovered that this oral solution had also a tonic effect in many people and so became aware that the magnesium chloride had an effect on the whole organism.

In a brief time, he received communications of very good therapeutic effects of this "therapy" from people that were taking magnesium chloride for its tonic properties and who were suffering from various ailments. Prof. Delbet began to closely study the subject and verified that the magnesium chloride solution was a very good therapy for a long list of diseases.

He obtained very good results in: inflammation of the colon (colitis), biliary vessels (angiocholitis), gall bladder (cholecystitis), in the digestive apparatus; Parkinson's Disease, senile tremors and muscular cramps, in the nervous system, acne, eczema, psoriasis, warts, itch of various origins and chilblains, in the skin. There was a strengthening of hair and nails, a good effect on diseases typical of the aged (impotency, prostatic hypertrophy, cerebral and circulatory troubles) and on diseases of allergic orgin (hay-fever, asthma, urticaria, and anaphylactic reactions).

Then Prof. Delbet began to investigate the relationship between magnesium and cancer. After a lot of clinical and experimental studies, he found that magnesium chloride had a very good effect on prevention of cancer and that it was able to cure several precancerous conditions: leucoplasia, hyperkeratosis, chronic mastitis, etc.

Epidemiological studies confirmed Delbet's views and demonstrated that the regions of soil with richer incidence of magnesium had less cancer, and vice versa.

In experimental studies, the magnesium chloride solution was also able to slow down the course of cancer in laboratory animals.

Prof. Delbert wrote two books, *Politique Preventive du Cancer* (1944) and *L'Agriculture et la Sante'* (1945), in which he stated his ideas about cancer prevention and a better living. The first is a well documented report of all his studies on magnesium chloride.

In 1943 another French doctor, Dr. A. Neveu, M.D., used the magnesium solution in a case of diptheria to reduce the risks of anaphylactic reaction due to the anti-diptheric serum that he was ready to administer. To his great surprise, when the next day the laboratory results confirmed the diagnosis of

34

diptheria, the little girl was completely cured before he could use the serum.

He credited the immuno-stimulant activity to the solution for this result, and he tested it in some other patients. All the patients were cured in a very short time (24 - 48 hours), with no after-effects.

Dr. Neveu then began to treat some cases of poliomyelitis, and had the same wonderful results. He was very excited and tried to divulge the therapy, but he ran into a wall of hostility and obstructionism from "official medicine." Neither Neveu or Delbet (who was a member of the Academy of Medicine) was able to diffuse Neveu's extraordinary results. The opposition was total: professors of Medicine, Medical peer-reviews, the Academy itself, all were against the two doctors. "Official medicine" saw in magnesium chloride therapy a threat to its new and growing business — vaccinations.

Dr. Neveu wasn't discouraged by this and continued to test this therapy in a wide range of diseases. He obtained very good results in: pharyngitis, tonsillitis, hoarseness, common cold, influenza, asthma, bronchitis, broncho-pneumonia, pulmonary emphysema, "children diseases" (whooping-cough, measles, rubella, mumps, scarlet fever . . .), alimentary and professional poisonings, gastroenteritis, boils, abscesses, localized inflammation and swelling of skin called erysipelas, draining inflammation at the end of a finger or a toe derived from within bone or under finger nail (whitlow), septic pricks (wounds), puerperal fever (fever during 3rd stage of labor) and inflammation of bone (osteomyelitis).

But the indications for magnesium chloride therapy don't end here. In more recent years other physicians, including Raul Vergini, M.D. of Italy, have verified many of Delbet's and Neveu's applications and have tried the therapy in other pathologies: asthmatic acute attack, shock, tetanus (for these the magnesium chloride is administered by intravenous injection); herpes zoster, acute and chronic inflammation of the eye (conjunctivitis), inflammation of the optic nerve (optic neuritis), rheumatic diseases, many allergic diseases, loss of strength (spring-asthenia), and chronic fatigue syndrome, (even in cancer it can be an useful coadjuvant.)

Dr. Vergini says, "The preceding lists of ailments are by no means exhaustive; maybe other illnesses can be treated with this therapy, but, as this is a relatively 'young' treatment, we are pioneers, and we need the help of all physicians of good will to definitely establish all the true possibilities of this wonderful therapy.

"From a practical standpoint, please remember that only magnesium chloride has this 'cytophilactic' activity, and no other magnesium salt; probably it's a molecular, and not a merely ionic, matter."[14]

The Magnesium Chloride Hexahydrate (MgCl2.6H2O) Solution According to Raul Vergini, M.D.

The solution to be used is a 2.5% magnesium chloride hexahydrate

(MgCl2.6H2O) solution (i.e.: 25 grams/liter of water).

Those who have kidney problems should be carefully monitored by their family physician, according to the Center for Disease Control. Dr. Raul Vergini says, that "this is true only for severe renal insufficiency, where an obvious contraindication may exist; but this is also true for all minerals that cannot be easily eliminated by a seriously impaired kidney. In all other cases, there are no risks. I never heard or read of any problem. The quantity of elemental magnesium contained in a 125 cc dose of the 2.5% solution is around 500 mg. That is not a large dose! Anyway, I think that it is a good precaution to advise people with renal problems to consult their physician."[14]

But Raul Vergini, M.D. also advises that "the problem is that very probably their physicians and pediatricians don't know anything about this therapy, so how can they give good advice? Children under 5, he says, nonetheless must consult their pediatrician."

Dosages are as follows:

Adults and children over 5 years old	125cc
4 year old children	100cc
3 year old children	80cc
1-2 year old children	60cc
over 6 months old children	30cc
under 6 months old children	15cc

These doses must be adminstered by mouth.

For chronic diseases, the standard treatment is one dose morning and evening for a long period.

In acute diseases the dose is administered every 6 hours (every 3 hours the first two doses if the case is serious); then space every 8 hours and then 12 hours as improvement goes on.

After recovery it's better going on with a dose every 12 hours for some days.

As a preventive measure, and as a magnesium supplement, one dose a day can be taken.

Magnesium Chloride, even if it's an inorganic salt, is very well absorbed and it's a very good supplemental magnesium source.

For intravenous injections, the formula is:

Magnesium Chloride Hexahydrate .	25 grams
Distilled Water	100 grams

Make injections of 10-20cc (over 10-20 minutes) once or twice a day.

Of course the solution must be sterilized.

According to Raul Vergini, M.D., "the 25% solution for IV injections is correct. Personally I never use it, I use only the oral way. But it was used over thirty years ago by some French doctors (5 grams in 20 ml of saline solution of distilled water) to treat tetanus and other less dangerous diseases (asthmatic attacks, choc, opthalmic herpes, herpes zoster, Quincke's oedema, itching, etc.). It was injected very slowly (in 10-20 minutes), and the results were very good.

"Moreover also the Myers' cocktail contains 2-5 ml of a 20% solution of magnesium chloride (along with other products that may contribute to make the solution more diluted). However, I think that if there are problems of 'burning' with the 25% concentration, it should be possible to use, with the same results, a 2.5% solution (the same used by mouth) by dissolving 5 grams of magnesium chloride in 200 ml of distilled water. The solution must be sterilized.

"The intramuscular way is not used because the solution is painful."

This therapy gives very good results also in veterinary medicine, at the appropriate dosages depending upon the size and kind of animals.

In the United States, magnesium chloride hexahydrate can be purchased chemically pure (c.p.) from most chemical supply houses without a prescription, although if you tell them why you're ordering this substance, they may feel compelled to "protect" you. Tell them it's for experimental purposes, or for your garden, or any reason that you find works.

Manganese Supplementation

Richard A. Kunin, M.D. of San Francisco, California, writes, "I've seen remarkable success in youngsters with cartilage hypertrophy and pain in the knees (so-called Osgood-Schlatter's disease), by administering manganese, another trace mineral in short supply."[23]

Molybdenum Supplementation

As reported by *The Alternative Medicine Digest*, British researcher Margaret Moss, M.A. conducted a study on the oral use of the essential micronutrient molybdenum over a 28 day period. Fourteen middle-aged people with symptoms of arthritis, low back pain, frozen shoulder, Rheumatoid Arthritis, and Osteoarthritis were given 400-500 mg daily (4-5 doses of 100 mg) of molybdenum amino acid chelate. "After 28 days, everyone on the trial felt better: toe and foot pain decreased, cramps and rheumatic pain declined, and the sense of well-being increased."[42]

According to Stephen Cooter, Ph.D. and Walter Schmitt, Jr., D.C., molydenum chelate converts ethanol and its descendents, aldehydes, produced by candida organisms into a substance that the body can use for energy, also removing the bad effects of the actyldehydes from tissues. It's speculatively reasonable to assume that some of the good benefits from molybdenum chelate supplementation derive from this fact. That is, many Fibromyalgia patients also probably suffer from candidiasis. (See "Candidiasis: Scourge of Arthritics" and "Molybdenum for *Candida albicans* Patients and Other Problems," http://www.arthritistrust.org.)

Juices and Filtered Water

Try drinking filtered water, apple cider vinegar, and eat honey on arising, before bed, and several times a day. Juice therapy can include equal parts of carrot, celery, cucumber and beet.[4]

Iron Supplements

Iron supplements may exacerbate various forms of arthritis, while flaxseed oil, essential fatty acids, and garlic may bring relief.[7] See *Iron: A Double Edged Sword.*"

Electro-Acuscope/Myopulse System of Therapy

Several electrical or "electronic" devices are used to reduce inflammation and pain in addition to the Light Beam Generator and Omega Ray reported in *Arthritis: Osteoarthritis and Rheumatoid Disease Including Rheumatoid Arthritis*, "Lymphatic Detoxification," "Lymph Drainage Therapy," http://www.arthritistrust.org.)

• The well-known TENS unit is intended to remove or reduce the patient's perception of pain.

• Galvanic stimulation produces muscle contraction and hence a strengthenintg effect.

• The Light Beam Generator produces a flow of pulsed negative electrons which temporarily liquifies poorly bound proteins, chiefly in the lymph system, permitting lymph to be more easily massaged out.

• The Electro-Acuscope/Myopulse system used by a trained practitioner is, like the Light Beam Generator, totally painless, but it operates in a different manner by inducing microcurrent stimulation of the proper frequency, intensity and duration to cause extracellular calcium ions to enter the cell through membrane pores (voltage-sensitive calcium ion channels). Higher levels of calcium then encourage increased synthesis of adenosine triphoshate (ATP), turning on mechanisms that control DNA and protein synthesis, thereby increasing the rate of cellular repair and replication.

This system also adjusts its waveform continuously in response to tissue impedance. This information is also reported to the therapist, who therefore can constantly monitor results.

The Electro-Acuscope, together with a Myopulse System, also addresses micro-acupuncture entry points along meridian lines that can enhance the functioning of internal organs at the same time.

Joan Shrum-Brown, Physical Therapist, owner/director of Marguerite Physical Therapy Clinic of Mission Viejo, California, feels that any condition involving nerve or muscle tissue can be improved, especially in conjunction

38

with "therapeutic exercise, body mechanics, and especially mobilization."

Physical therapist Shrum-Brown uses the system most frequently for patients with muscle spasms, temporomandibular joint disorders, Bursitis, arthritis, surgical incisions, sprains and strains, herpes zoster infections, dysmenorrhea and hematomas."[47]

According to Mark Kana, Physical Therapist, supervisor of physical therapy for Southwest General hospital and its Sports West Clinic in Middleburg Heights, Ohio, "the best response depends not on the specific diagnosis, but on the skill of the user. The modality's applications are limited only when the user is not employing the full spectrum of treatment."[47]

Over the the past three years, Mark Kana, P.T. uses the Electro-Acuscope/ Myopulse system to treat a variety of conditions involving the neck, back, hip, knee, ankle, and shoulder.

Where the Light Beam Generator requires about 20 minutes to treat a sprained ankle, the Electro-Acuscope/Myopulse system requires about 3 minutes. Herm Schneider, A.T.C., Head Athletic Trainer for the Chicago White Sox, is reported as saying that "We have just about excluded ice and the routine treatments for sprains and bruises, and we treat players immediately as they come out of the game."

The Case of Bo Jackson

Bo Jackson was signed by the White Sox as a free agent before the 1991 season after he was released by the Kansas City Royals.

Gary Emerson, D.C., Santa Ana, California, consultant for many well-known sports figures, at the request of White Sox's Herm Schneider, A.T.C., used the Electro-Acuscope as part of Jackson's rehabilitation, and Bo appeared in 23 games with the White Sox.

After undergoing hip replacement surgery in 1992, Bo was treated with the Electro-Acuscope immediately afterward to speed recovery.

The Case of Paul Asmuth

Reported by Godfrey, marathon swimmer Paul Asmuth sought aid for myositis (inflammation of the muscle) and capsulitis (inflammation of the capsule) of the shoulder only days before a 21-mile marathon swim that included a punishing final stretch against the tide. "After five Electro-Acuscope/Myopulse treatments Asmuth was able to outdistance a swimmer ten years his junior, finishing second and providing how rapidly his shoulder condition had improved."

Electro-Acuscope's Range of Uses

The Electro-Acuscope can be used for acute and chronic pain mainly of musculoskeletal origin: automobile accidents, lumbrosacral sprains, shoulder strains, rotator cuff tears, and sports injuries. Others have used it for herpes zoster neuralgia, local skin infections, bedsores, spasticity, chronic fatigue syndrome, migraine and other headaches, and also for Carpal Tunnel Syndrome.

Jerry Fisher, President of Electron-Medical Incorporated, manufacturers and distributors of the Electro-Acuscope, writes that "An arthritis diagnosis is quite often a 'catch-all' diagnosis. The doctors use this diagnosis when there is pain around a joint and they don't know the cause. In most cases, the pain is soft tissue inflammation or muscle injury that can be treated with the Electro-Acuscope. It is very common for one or two treatments to completely solve the pain. . . . In conditions where it may actually be arthritis, such as pain in finger joints, it is usually just as easy to treat. Even when heat can be felt in the painful joint, you can feel the temperature return to normal in a few minutes of treating and the pain will go away at the same time."[48]

The Photon Sound Beam

This instrument utilizes similar gas tube technology to that of the Light Beam Generator or Electro-Acuscope, and also affects the lymph system in a manner similar to the Light Beam Generator. Inert or noble gases contained in round glass tubes are evacuated of air and filled, under pressure, with Argon and Xenon. A high voltage at low current ionizes the gases to a plasma state.

Two glass photon tubes with insulated handles are included in each unit. A high voltage energy is produced by an electronic circuit that derives the energy by means of a pulse repetition rate in the audio spectrum. According to a spokesperson for the Sunshine Company, Ogden, Utah, "This pulse rate has been proven over a long period of time to be of benefit to the human body, as a form of energy, much like normal exercise."[57]

A small black box, "RF Sound Probe," is also provided that produces an additional "receiving glass electrode," and is to be used together with the other glass electrodes.

Full instructions on its use are also provided with each instrument.

The Omega Ray

The Omega Ray operates very much like the Light Beam Generator (See *Lymphatic Detoxification*, and *Lymph Drainage* at http://www.arthritistrust.org) with the additional ability to generate a random pattern or varying cycle of frequencies. The advantage of this randomness is that it is believed that the body will be less likely to accomodate or become resistant to the energy.

Environmental Factors (Clinical Ecology)

Harold Buttram, M.D.,[45] Woodlands Medical Center, Quakertown, Pennsylvania, writes that "I have a number of toxicology and environmental texts, but not one of them mentions fire-retardants. It would appear that mattress manufactureers are very guarded about the chemicals that they use. I can understand why, since some of them may be quite toxic." (See "Our Toxic World: Who's Looking After Our Kids?" http://www.arthritistrust.org.)

The Case of Judith Tolbett

A 59 year old lady presented herself to the office of Harold Buttram,

40

M.D. with complaints of muscle pains of 3 years duration. Dr. Buttram describes Judith's symptoms: "The onset of the pains occurred abruptly and rapidly progressed to the point that she could barely move her arms and legs. She was referred to a hematologist who diagnosed polymyalgia rheumatica (rheumatoid pains in many muscles) based on clinical findings and an elevated sedimentation rate. In addition an antinuclear antibody test was positive.

"During the interview in our office the patient was questioned about possible chemical exposures, especially solvent-type of fumes such as those arising from fresh indoor painting, pesticides, new wall-to-wall carpets, disinfectant cleaning solutions, and other possible sources. At first the patient could not recall any exposures, but towards the end of the interview she remembered that she had purchased a new mattress shortly before the onset of her illness. She related that the matress had a strong, unpleasant chemical smell, so unpleasant that her husband refused to sleep on it and moved to another room. In spite of this Judith continued sleeping on the mattress.

"When it was pointed out to Judith that volatile organic compounds, all of which are potentially toxic, are often impregnated into matresses as fire retardants or preservatives, there was a dawning realization on her part that the unpleasant smell could have been the underlying cause of the illness. I was convinced that this was the case."

In the view of Dr. Buttram, "The major lesson to be derived from this case rests in the fact that if she had been seen by a physician trained in environmental medicine at or near the onset of her illness rather than 3 years later, and if the toxic volatile chemical exposure had been recognized as the cause of her illness and therefore avoided, the more serious complications of her illness might have been avoided."

According to Harold Buttram, M.D. "As is often the case in environmental illnessess caused by chemical exposures, implication of volatile chemical exposure as a cause of the illness was based on circumstantial evidence. Laboratory tests which might have been helpful at time of Judith's onset of muscle pain would be useless after a lapse of 3 years. However, there were ample clinical grounds for assuming a high degree of probability that breathing the fumes over a prolonged period of time did cause the illness.

"First, there was the time factor with the onset of severe illness in a previously healthy woman soon after exposures to the noxious fumes.

"Second, scientific studies have shown that occupational or home exposures to volatile organic compounds such as formaldehyde, chlorinated and organophosphate pesticides, trichlorethylene and other halogenated hydrocarbons, toluene diisoccyanate, and trimellitic anhydride cause significant increases of autoantibodies to smooth muscles, parietal (cavity) cells, brushborder cells (ciliated cells lining nasal passages, bronchial tubes, and the small intestines), and mitochondria. These auto-antibodies probably form the basis for myalgic (muscle) pains commonly seen in environmental illness. The involvement of the mitochondria, which provide the major source of body energy, probably explains why fatigue is almost invariably a major symptom in environmental illness.

"Although well-intentioned, there is a federal law requiring fire-retardants in mattresses." As Dr. Buttram understands the law, "a doctor's prescription is required for purchasers wishing to avoid these chemicals. Unfortunately the law does not proscribe the use of potentially dangerous chemicals or require the use of safer forms of fire-retardants and preservatives."

Treatment According to Harold Buttram, M.D.

The field of chemical detoxification is a vast one with a variety of approaches. In order to achieve wellness, Judith Tolbett was provided with regimens and advice by Dr. Buttram, which follow:

Avoid Chemicals: "As with all such cases, first emphasis for Judith was placed on the avoidance of chemical exposures. As an educated guess, perhaps 75 or 80% of treatment for environmental illness involves this avoidance, without which the best of conventional and/or alternative treatment will fail. Naturally the first recommendation was for her to replace the mattress with one without fire-retardants or chemical preservatives, consisting of natural materials (not foam rubber). Beyond this she was provided with educational materials concerning common sources of dangerous chemicals in the home and workplace and the use of safe alternatives.

"Once an individual has been sensitized or made ill by chemical exposures, each additional exposure further weakens the body, since the effects tend to be cumulative. Consequently first emphasis should be placed on education of the patient as to common sources of dangerous chemicals in the home, school, or workplace and the use of safe alternatives.

"For physician education, Dr. Buttram suggests the American Academy of Environmental Medicine, 4510 W. 89th Street, Prairie Village, Kansas 66207; (913) 642-6062.

Diet: "Special emphasis was placed on chemical-free, largely vegetarian diet, organically grown as much as practicable, since such a diet tends to be anti-inflammatory.

"For nutritional supplements Judith was given flax seed oil capsules (high in anti-inflammatory Omega-3 fatty acids), barley juice powder (high in chlorophyll, also a potent anti-inflammatory agent), a thymus glandular tablet as an immune stimulant, and glucosamine sulfate (to restore joint cartilage).

"On this program the patient showed marked improvement after about a month, but unfortunately, when under a great deal of stress during a terminal illness of her mother, she developed a fever and had a relapse of her symptoms."

According to Dr. Buttram's case summary, "The tragedy of this case is

42

that the true nature and cause of this patient's illness was not recognized in its early stages. If the real culprit in her illness, that of toxic chemical exposure, had been recognized and removed, in all likelihood she would have had a short illness followed by complete recovery. As is evident from her subsequent course, there is some degree of permanent damage resulting in a fragile state of health."

Antioxidant Vitamins: The oxidative system is supported by antioxidant vitamins such as vitamins C and E. beta carotene, and pycnogenol, and by the minerals magnesium, zinc, copper, manganese, and selenium. Various herbs can also be used such as milk thistle seed, dandelion root, beet root, black radish, and golden seal root. There are many others.

According to Harold Buttram, M.D. "It should be pointed out that detoxification of xenobiotic chemicals (volatile organic compounds) takes place largely in the liver by the action of two enzyme systems. The first is the cytochrome P450 oxidase system which, by the process of <u>oxidation</u>, brings about alteration of the xenobiotics from their fat or lipid-soluble state to a more water soluble state in which they are more toxic than its parent compound. Consequently, in health it is instantly bound or disarmed by the process of <u>conjugation</u>, a process in which the enzyme glucuronidase is a major actor. If either of these two systems is crippled or overburdened, as is commonly the case in environmental illness, then xenobiotic chemicals accumulate in the body."

Conjugation: The conjugation process which disarms toxic substances is supported or "fed" by such supplements as blue-green algae, garlic, reduced glutathione, taurine, and methionine. These provide sources of sulfhydryl groups utilized in the conjugation phase of detoxification.

Other treatment regimens, tests and procedures used by Dr. Buttram may include:

Salt Water Baths, Saunas and Aerobic Exercises: These have the common goal of mobilizing xenobiotic chemicals from fat stores in the body and their elimination through sweat. We have found that epsom salt baths conducted in the patient's home are often preferable because of convenience and lack of expense to the patient. We instruct the patient to add 2 pounds of epsom salt to a hot tub and then soak for 20 to 30 minutes every other day. Regarding aerobic exercise, it should be followed immediately by a bath or shower so that chemicals will not be reabsorbed through the open pores. (See "Allergies and Biodetoxification for the Arthritic," http://www.arthritistrust.org.)

Other Supplements: Dr. Buttram suggests that one might also include niacin, olive oil (Virgin), flax seed oil, choline and inositol, all of which have the purpose of mobilizing and eliminating xenobiotic chemicals. It should be cautioned that niacin, which stimulates release of xenobiotics from fat tissues, can cause liver damage in higher doses.

Laboratory Tests: Dr. Buttram has found the following tests useful: hair

43

test for minerals and toxic heavy metals, red blood cell mineral analysis, functional vitamin analysis, urine or blood amino acids, liver detoxification panel, volatile hydrocarbon panels (if exposures have been recent), autoimmune and chemical antibodies in selected cases.

Individualization of Therapies: Dr. Buttram says that "As is always the case in medicine, best results are obtained when the therapy is tailored to the individual patient. This requires some familiarity by the physician with the field of environmental medicine. Considering the prevalence of environmental illness today, should not all physicians gain some familiarity with this field? The basics are not difficult!"

Enzyme Therapy

Enzyme supplementation, along with proper diet, may be a key to getting well.

The Case of Oscar Hernandez[53]

Oscar Hernadez was a 26-year-old wealthy sufferer of polymyositis, a condition where inflammation is found in many muscles. When Hector Solorzano del Rio, M.D., Ph.D., D.Sc. met Oscar in San Miguel Allende, a small town in Mexico, Oscar had already visited some of the best rheumatologists in San Antonio, Texas, La Jolla, California, and Rochester, Minnesota.

Oscar had been placed on the fantastic dosage of 250 mg of corticosteroids for four months and during that interval the side-effects had destroyed his ability to walk, created diarrhea, digestive problems, and collapsed his right lung so that he couldn't breathe.

Dr. Hector Solorazono del Rio first explained to Oscar that if he were to get well he'd have to change his life style, eating habits and attitude toward life. Then Dr. Solorzano used the Dermatron — a device that measures bio-electric energy along meridian acupuncture lines — to determine the proper diet for Oscar, which diet Hernandez was placed on for two months. During this period Oscar was given intravenous infusions of dimethylsulfoxide (DMSO) and cocarboxylase.

According to Susana Alcazar Leyva, vice president of the Hans Selye Institute of Scientific Research, San Jeronimo, Mexico, D.F., and president of the Albert Szent-Gyorgyi, Gerontological Center, Tlacote 128, Juriquilla 76320, the coenzyme cocarboxylase (thiamin pyrophosphate: TPP) improves metabolism, and provides good effects at the neural and hormonal level, as demonstrated in clinical and experimental investigations.

"Hair mineral analysis, when done properly, can provide information on 27 normal minerals and 7 toxic heavy metals," Dr. Solorzano reports, and based on these tests, Oscar was determined to have high levels of lead and arsenic. Dr. Solorzano chelated out these toxic metals, using EDTA chelation therapy. (See "Chelation Therapy," http://www.arthritistrust.org.)

Dr. Solorzano also advised Oscar to take a number of the traditional anti-oxidants, as well as the essential fatty acids "which," he says, "is usually low in most arthritic patients."

Oscar Hernandez could walk again after two months of treatment.

After six months of treatment, Dr. Solorazano started Hernandez on enzyme therapy.

After 9 months of treatment, Oscar was completely well. In a letter to Dr. Solorzano he wrote, "After this period of time, I find myself with health 100%. I've returned to normal and I now swim 1000 meters daily, lift weights, and am in excellent health. My mood is also excellent. The only limitations I have remaining are diminished strength in my hands, but I expect to solve this soon."[53]

Herbs

Based on the clinical experience of 150 patients over a 4-year period, Brent W. Davis, D.C.[56] says that "I have seen Cat's Claw break through severe intestinal derangements that no other product can touch," including diverticulitis, recurring ulcers, Crohn's disease, irritable and leaky bowel syndrome, and depressed intestinal action. Cat's Claw is also useful in clearing up long-term parasitic infestations in the intestines involving *Balstocystis hominis*, *entamoebas*, and *Giardia*.

Cat's Claw, trademarked as SAVENTARO^{TM}, is a standardized, pharmaceutical grade, expiration dated, ecologically farmed root compound from *Uncaria tomentosa*, a creeping shrub native to the Peruvian rainforest. Extracts from this plant have long been used in Amazonian tribal medicine.

In 1959, Dr. Klaus Keplinger, an Austrian doctor, was introduced to the beneficial qualities of the root of the plant by a respected Amazonian shaman who urged Dr. Keplinger to share this knowledge with the world. The first samples were analyzed at the University of Innsruck, and since then both European and American scientists have been investigating the effects and therapeutic applications of the *Uncaria tomentosa* plant. Several patents have been awarded to Dr. Klepinger for his research findings, and, after 25 years of research and clinical trials, Dr. Keplinger and his daughter Ursula Keplinger, have both dedicated themselves to fulfilling the wishes of the Ashaninca shaman.

Root material is gathered in the ecological farm set up jointly with Immodal Pharmaka in 1988. Collections are made in such a way as to preserve the rainforest.

It is important to note that only the root has strong beneficial qualities, although others on the market use an inferior portion of the vine, also often to the detriment of the vine.

Immodal Pharmaka, an Austrian firm that produces SAVENTARO, founded in 1989, has sold the product for use in allergic diseases, herpes infections, Rheumatoid Arthritis, carcinomas, weak immunological system, and for HIV infections.[46]

(See Peruvian Rainforest Botanicals online.)

From 1983 to 1985, six patients suffering from Rheumatoid Arthritis participated in trial therapy. During the first controlled treatment cycle the patients were given 60 ml of SAVENTARO tea every day, this being the equivalent to 3 mg alkaloids daily. Four of the six patients subsequently continued with the test preparation using capsules. The daily dosage was equivalent to 20 mg to 60 mg SAVANTARO extract daily.

During the first three months three of the six patients complained of increased pain while the other three experienced a lessening of such pain as early as the first month.

Six months later all patients reported a lessening of pain and reduction of inflammation plus improved movement. Reduction in blood sedimentation rate was a striking benefit. Good clinical health was maintained by patients on an average of 1.7 to 5.7 years without need for further therapy.

After an intervening period of 9.2 years (average), all of these patients were questioned regarding the long-term effects of the treatment.

After 12 months, 3 of the patients were largely free of pain while the other 3 still suffered from reduced pain, although they had experienced some pain-free intervals.

After 18 months all patients were largely no longer suffering any pain.

Unfortunately this test was made with simultaneous use of damaging gold salts, non-steroidal anti-inflammatory drugs, and the use of cortisone when required. So SAVANTERO is most likely more beneficial taken without these damaging products, and the actual independent effects of the compound are still to be ascertained.

This same root compound, with the name of Krallendorn, is sold in Europe under Austrian and German health authorities for treatment of arthritis.

According to Davis' report in *Alternative Medicine Digest*,[56] Cat's Claw can be administered in the range of 3-25 g daily, in tear or tablet form. As a liquid extract, Dr. Davis usually gives it at the rate of 3 g daily, or 25 drops 3 times daily, normally not to exceed 5 g daily during an initial 10-14 day period.

Garlic (*Allium sativum*) has been widely used throughout the world for centuries, for a variety of conditions, among which is its use for Rheumatism. "Garlic and its prepartions are known for their antibiotic, antifungal, and anti-viral activity."[4]

Nettle (*Urtica dioica*), is widely used in the Western world. "If used regularly over the long-term it can be remarkably successful in cases of Rheumatism and arthritis."[4]

"Combine the tinctures of meadowsweet, horsetail, and willow bark in equal parts and take one teaspoonful three times a day. Topically either gently rub into the affected area a mixture of equal parts tincture of lobelia and cramp bark to the effected muscles. Drink strong chamomile tea, particularly at bed-time to help relieve pain. Aloe vera gel may be helpful."[4]

Leon Chaitow, D.O., provides a herbal combination formula to be used as a tonic that "will support people with chronic weakness, anxiety, head-aches, sleep disturbances and general fatigue, as well as diminished blood flow to the extremeties. A person who needs this will probably have a weak pulse, weak digestive system, headaches and be fatigued."[8]

Mix 2 parts each of *Panax quinquefolium* (American ginseng), *Astragalus monoglicus*, and *Angelica sinensis* (dong quai); 1 part each of *Cimicifuga racemosa* (black cohosh), and *Passiflora incarnata* (passion flower); with 1/2 part each of *Betonica officinalis* (wood betony); *Matricaria chamomila* (chamomile), and *Zizyphus sativa* (jujube red dates). Between one-half and one teaspoon, two or three times weekly, taken between meals is suggested.[8]

Dr. Chaitow also suggests using *Ginkgo biloba* more with treatment of Fibromyalgia and chronic fatigue syndrome.[8]

Antonio Ruiz, M.D. of San Antonio, Texas, reported that "many patients with a variety of stress-induced soft-tissue pain conditions such as Fibrositis and occupational cumulative trauma disorders are reporting substantial relief with *Boswellia serrata*.[13]

As many Fibromyalgia patients have difficulty sleeping, David Squires, a Fibromyalgia sufferer, recommends Valerian Rest[TM] with lemon balm. He writes, "Numerous scientific studies confirm valerian's efficacy in relieving in-somnia and improving the quality of sleep. . . .Valerian root is a safe and proven sleep aid." Valerian Rest[TM] is non-addictive and leaves no groggi-ness and contains lemon balm which has historically been used to treat ner-vous anxiety, insomnia, depression, and indigestion.[24]

Feverfew is combined with rosemary and cayenne in a substance called Feverfew Formula[TM] by David Squires. "The principal component in fever-few is called parthenolide, and it inhibits the production of certain prostaglan-dins, (as would the proper essential fatty acids and diet) including leukotrienes (slow-reacting substances that stimulate allergic reactions) and amines (a sub-stance known to increase in the brain during migraine attacks)." In Squires formulation the rosemary and the cayenne act together enhancing the pain-relieving properties.[24]

Cayenne pepper, capsicum or chili pepper, is related to the potato-to-mato family, the solanines. The chemical responsible for the hotness of this pepper and its medicinal effects is capsaicin (cap-SAY-shun) . Pure capsaicin has been the subject of most intensive research and has been proven effec-tive for pain relief.

For over twenty-five years studies have shown that capsaicin can reduce sensitivity in pain caused by heat, pressure, and chemicals.

Since somewhere between 30 and 50% of arthritics have a chemical sensitivity to the solanines, caution is advised when relying on capsaicin.

Alan Gaby, M.D.[16] reported on a study consisting of forty-five patients with Fibromyalgia. A 0.025% capsaicin cream (from *Capsicum frutescens*) or a placebo 4 times daily were rubbed on tender areas in a double blind study. After four weeks, capsaicin-treated patients had significantly less tenderness at their tender points then did placebo patients, and a significant increase in grip strength was observed after two weeks in the capsaicin group. Dr. Gaby writes that "Capsaicin works by depleting substance P, a mediator of pain in afferent nerve fibers. Although this treatment is not a cure, it is relatively safe, and is worth considering for Fibromyalgia patients."

David Squires writes, "I had tried capsaicin in the past and didn't think it worked on my pain. He (David's doctor) convinced me to try again by explaining that because it was a topical and a natural ingredient, it took time to work. It had to be put on several times a day and over an extended period of time before I would see results. . . . Fibromyalgia patients have up to three times more substance-P than the normal person. So I faithfully applied it for four weeks and was ready to give up again when I felt pain relief for the first time without side effects like stomach upsets, toxicity, or addiction." As Capsaicin was expensive, David searched around for other products, finding at last aloe vera based gel with the same concentration of capsaicin as the product he had started with, but at a fraction of the cost. The substance was Pain-Free ^{TM}. David says, "not only did it help Fibromyalgia pain, but many different kinds of chronic pain such as Osteoarthritis and Rheumatoid Arthritis, neuralgias, and diabetic neuropathy."[24]

Fibromyalgia, neuralgia and minor muscle strains are all candidates for the use of capsaicin, but keep in mind that repeated applications are necessary as substance-P does not disappear overnight. Effective use of the capsaicin cream, according to Julie Nowak,[42] requires topical application 2-3 times daily for a period of at least 4 weeks. "A phyotomedicine containing 0.075% capsaicin in a cream base is available in a high-potency but for most people, the lower percent of capsaicin works just as well."

A herbal tea with long staying power is Kombucha Tea. Dr. L. Mollenda wrote in 1928 that Kombucha beverage "proved itself effective especially in troubles of the digestive organs, whose function it completely normalized. In addition, the beverage proved itself effective in cases of Gout, Rheumatism, and various stages of arteriosclerosis."[37]

The use of yucca plant extracts are an ancient American Indian remedy. The yucca extract contains a saponin (soapy emulsifier) and a safe, vegetable steroid, according to Robert Bingham, M.D., who used yucca plant extract for many years on his patients to improve arthritic conditions. According to

Dr. Bingham when yucca food supplements are taken two to three times a day, "its action improves digestion and elimination and reduces harmful bacteria in the intestines. This is reflected in the relief of joint pains and stiffness. An unexpected discovery has been reduced fat levels in the blood. Circulation is improved, and blood flows more freely through the muscles and joints... [an important benefit for Fibromyalgia patients]. No toxic or harmful effects of yucca extract have been found in treating thousands of patients over more than ten years.... the use of yucca food supplements ... is beneficial in 80-90%, reducing joint pain and stiffness."[54]

As reported in *Alternative Medicine: The Definitive Guide*, boil three to four mullein leaves in water for three minutes, placing the pack over the painful joint. Wrap it with a hot, moist towel, then a dry towel, leaving it for twenty minutes three times a day.[4]

Homeopathy

According to Leon Chaitow, D.O., *Rhus toxicodendron* (Rhus tox), a homeopthic remedy, has shown both good results and poor results in Fibromyalgia and Fibrositis studies, depending upon the strength used. A high potency solution (very low concentration, 6C dilution) was found effective in trials in Britain, but a lower potency (high concentration 6X dilution) was found ineffective in Australia.[8]

It must be clearly understood that homeopathic remedies, and their potencies, are determined by the individual's characteristics. A physical, constitutional, and personality profile of the patient is identified, matched against "proven" remedies, and then only those particular remedies at their concentrations are to be used.[8]

Dr. Andrew Lockie, author of *The Family Guide to Homeopathy*, writes: "All homeopathic remedies have a double personality. On the one hand they are known to *cause* a range of symptoms in perfectly healthy people. On the other hand, by the law of similars, they are known to *alleviate* the same symptoms in people who are unwell. However remedies that match physical symptoms only may not be enough to provoke a return to health. Ideally, to provide the greatest healing, a remedy should match the physical symptoms, the mental symptoms, and the constitution of the person concerned."[32]

When 24 double-blinded patients presented symptoms that matched the proper selection of *Arnica*, *Bryonia* and *Rhus Toxicodendron* (Rhus Tox), and were given one of the three remedies, results showed a statistically significant improvement.[31]

According to *Alternative Medicine: The Definitive Guide*, for Fibroymalgia use *Belladonna, Arnica, Ruta graveolens, Silicea*.[4]

Dr. Schuessler's Biochemistry[27] reports on the use of the mineral salts as follows:

• *Ferrum phosphorus* is to be used for pain, fever, heat, redness and quickened pulse in the first stages of rheumatism.

• *Kali muriate* should be used during the Fibrositis, or second stage of Rheumatism, when swelling has resulted. The tongue will be thick, white or have a greying coating, and when movement increases pain, and there is swelling of the joints. *Kali muriate* can be alternated with *Ferrum phosphorus.*

Natrum phosphorus is a principal remedy when there is sour-smelling perspiration or acid conditions, with an acid taste in the mouth and creamy-yellow coating on the base of the tongue.

Kali sulphuricum is useful when the pains shift suddenly from place to place, and when pains worsen in a heated room or in the evening, yet feel better in cool air.

Kali phosphorus is used when there is stiffness of the joints or when associated with nervous conditions, and also when pains worsen on starting to move, but are relieved by continual, gentle motion.

Natrum muriate is used when there is characteristic watery discharge of joints, and they worsen at night, in bad weather with heat, cold or change of weather, or when one has cold sensations.

Calcarea Phosphorus is for Rheumatism that is worse at night and in bad weather, heat or cold, dampness and change of weather, and when there is stiffness and numbness of the joints.

Calcarea fluor is used when there is enlargement of the joints.

Magnesia phosphorus is for acute, sharp spasmodic pains, or excruciating, violent pains relieved by warmth.

Silicea is for pains in the shoulders that worsen at night and from warm covering.

According to Dr. Andrew Lockie,[32] in Fibrositis, those small adhesions between individual muscle fibers that cause pain and stiffness usually clear up in 3 to 4 days provided muscles haven't been torn. The specific remedies that should be considered to be taken every 3 hours for up to 2 days are:

Aconite 30c used when "pain comes on suddenly in cold dry weather and seems to be aggravated by movement," and the person is restless and apprehensive.

Arnica 30c used, "When the muscles are bruised, as if from sleeping on a bed that is too hard, when movement makes pain worse, and the person has physical restlessness and irritability."

Bryonia 30c used when there is Fibrositis in the neck, back, and limbs, and it is made worse by movement and by dry, cold, east winds, soothed by pressure.

Causticum 6c for aching, tearing pains in limb muscles, with stiffness or weakness and the pain wears off in warm, wet weather, but gets worse in cold.

Chamomilla 6c used for pain and stiffness, having to get up in the night

50

because of the pain, and feeling bad tempered as if nothing is going right.

Ledum 6c used when the affected muscles feel cold but pain and stiffness is relieved by cold applications.

Nux 6c used when the pain and stiffness worsen in damp weather, in cold, dry weather, after exercise and around 4 a.m., when turning over in bed hurts, pressure brings on some relief, and the person is feeling irritable.

Rhus toxicodendron (Rhus Tox) 6c for muscles stiff after overuse, and the stiffness improves with gentle movement, and when the person is restless.

Additional suggestions by Dr. Lockie to accompany use of the above remedies is to take hot baths and apply hot and cold compresses alternately to stimulate circulation.

For Bursitis, Dr. Lockie[72] recommends, to be taken 4 times daily for up to 7 days:

Apis 30c when burning, stinging pain is made worse by heat.

Rhus toxicondendron 6c when tearing pain, joint stiffness and swelling is made worse by rest and cold, damp weather, alleviated by heat and gentle exercise.

Pulsatilla 6c when dragging pain and tightness is over the bursa and discomfort worsens when affected limb is allowed to hang, and there is general chilliness.

Sticta 6c for shooting pains.

Kali Iod. 6c when pains worsen at night.

Bryonia 30c when pain is made worse by heat or the slightest movement.

Belladonna 30c when pain is made worse by the slightest jarring, the joint is red, hot, and swollen and throbbing.

Ruta 6c when there is housemaid's knee, pain in thigh when knee is straightened, or a joint that feels bruised and weak.

Hormone Therapy

As multiple enzyme deficiencies (Wilson's syndrome) can display with more than 60 symptoms, including those accompanying Bursitis and Fibromyalgia, hormonal replacement therapy or other corrective hormonal therapy should be given serious consideration. (See "Thyroid Therapy: Cutting the Gordian Knot," http://www.arthritistrust.org.)

Hydrotherapy

Use alternating hot and cold packs one to three times daily to relieve pain, and stimulate blood flow. According to Leon Chaitow, N.D., D.O., ". . . any hot treatment (or bath) should finish with the area being chilled by a compress or spray (shower)."[4] If pain is acute, apply an ice pack twenty minutes out of each hour for the first twenty-four to thirty-six hours.

According to *Alternative Medicine: The Definitive Guide*,[4] soak for twenty-five to thirty minutes, using a pound or more of Epsom salts per bath. Rinse and rub down with hot olive oil, and do so once a week. Also rosemary soaks can be used for hands and feet or one might bathe the whole body by soaking for ten to fifteen minutes, two to three times a day.

If ice packs are preferred, place one above joint and one below for twenty minutes three times a day for one month."[8]

Iron Overload

Veterinarian Leslie N. Johnston, D.V.M.[28] believes that there is good reason to check every Fibromyalgia patient for iron overload.

In a rheumatology clinic in Australia, 339 patients were studied over a 12 month period of time. Twenty three patients had unusually high indices of iron — transferrin saturation and ferritin. Twelve of twenty of these patients who were measured again under fasting conditions showed elevated results "consistent with genetic iron overload (hemochromatosis)," which can cause a variety of illnesses, including cirrhosis of the liver, bronze skin pigmentation, diabetes mellitus, heart problems (cardiomyopathy presented as cardiomegaly), heart failure, and heart rhythm or conduction disturbances, pituitary failure, abdominal pain, arthritis, chondrocalcinosis, testicular atrophy and loss of libido."

Dr. Johnston also reports that cattle, horses, monkeys (Lemurs) and mynah birds are all capable of suffering from iron overload, as well as man.

Two solutions to a potential overload problem is (1) to donate blood, thus reducing your total iron content; (2) be chelated with desoferroxamine, a substance capable of combining with iron radicals found in tissues, and removing them through the urine. Iron bound to protein in blood is not at all dangerous, but healthy. When iron becomes free to bind with other tissues not intended to be bound with iron, the condition can be unhealthy.

Note that females have a natural way of eliminating excessive iron while males do not.

Magnetic Therapy

If there is one therapy that is universal, low cost and effective it is the use of magnets applied at the right place in the correct manner.

Physcists are taught that there is no difference between applying the positive or negative side of the magnet to your tissue because they discern no difference in using magnets to attract or repel in their laboratory. The definitive experiment demonstrating otherwise anyone one can do for themself. Tape a small magnet of the North seeking pole to your arm and leave it there for several weeks. When you remove the magnet you'll find redness, perhaps swelling, maybe even some infection. Now tape the South seeking side to your arm. After several weeks you'll find a healthy appearing skin and certainly zero infection.

Both sides of the magnet when used to kill pain will do so, but in entirely differen t ways. The North seeking side will increase endorphins leading some to become hooked on their own endorphins. The South seeking side will

52

change your tissues from acidic to alkaline, a must for anyone attempting to achieve wellness.

Standing on the broad shoulders of Albert Roy Davis, Robert O. Becker, G. Sheldon, Otto Warburg and others, William Philpott, psychiatrist and medical doctor extraordinary, has confirmed and extended their scientific work on the relationship of magnets to human biology. He presents in his book *The Magic of Magnetic Healing* (Amazon.com) a lifetime of experiences that clearly demonstrate the fundamentals of achieving wellness as well as documentation and instruction on how you can overcome that "impossible" medical problem. It's rare to find a doctor who is sufficiently open minded to be willing to look beyond cookbook remedies.

Medicine as it is presently practiced is all about buying patented chemicals that hopefully will jog the body into at least hiding symptoms if nothing else. Here Philpott demonstrates the basic underlying problem common to almost all disease states -- and he further clearly shows how to use that knowledge to turn about even the most complex health problems. Except for the stomach, bodily tissues should be alkaline and loaded with oxygen. Magnets do this for you and also kill microorganisms bringing about wellness, it appears, no matter how severe is the medical problem. William H. Philpott, M.D. has developed excellent treatment protocols and magnets for treating a wide range of diseases and pain conditions. There's no question of magnetic energy's ability to reduce pain. What is not so well known is that the polarity of the magnetics used can enhance healing or inhibit healing. Dr. Philpott has described numerous cases of not just pain relief, but also cures of otherwise "incurable" problems. He's also identified many physiological functions that are affected by magnetism, too numerous to mention here.

The definition of magnetic polarity used by Dr. Philpott is that of an electrical definition of polarity, which is positive and negative. This is purposely used when applying magnets to the human body rather than the navigational definition of magnetism as north seeking and south seeking.

The human body functions on a direct current circuit and thus, references to positive and negative are most appropriate. A positive electric field produces a positive magnetic field. A negative electric field produces a negative magnetic field. This parallel makes it possible to appropriately use the electric terms of polarity.

It has been recommended that it is preferred to use the electric definition of polarity instead of navigational definition of polarity when referring to magnetic polarity. An important point of referring to the separateness of the two magnetic poles is that the biological response is opposite to the separate poles. Some have elected to use a positive magnetic field of a combined positive-negative magnetic fields of low level gauss strength which serves as a counterirritant. However, the limitations of this is such as to not recommend this type of stress reflex therapy. It is more appropriate to have a higher gauss strength and use the negative magnetic pole for its anti-inflammatory value.

Some have also elected to use a pulsing frequency associated with a magnetic pole. Although this can be useful, it is not necessary.

What we have described in this article is a static magnetic field plus a pulsing field. The brain makes a pulsing response to the magnetic field it receives. When increasing the positive magnetic field the brain frequency increases and the amplitude decreases. When the brain is exposed to a negative magnetic field the brain frequency decreases and the amplitude increases.

The resting brain has a pulsing frequency of 8 to 12 cycles per second. This is a response to the negative magnetic field.

Sleep has runs as low as 2 cycles per second, which cycles per second is anti-stressful.

Any pulsing frequency above 12 cycles per second is stressful. Any pulsing frequency below 12 cycles is anti-stressful. The pulsing frequencies can be used for their value separate from a magnetic field or combined with a magnetic field. However, since the brain makes its own pulsing frequency response to the magnetic field there is no essential necessity of associating a pulsing frequency with the magnetic field.

This is truly a magnetic resonance therapy.

It is an oxidative therapy by virtue of the increase in oxygen that occurs under the influence of a negative magnetic field. A positive magnetic field would decrease the content of oxygen in the tissues under the influence of that positive magnetic polarity.

The pH Factor

Acute reactions to foods, chemicals, and inhalants are all acidifying.

Chronic reactions that become diagnosed as chronic degenerative diseases are simply extensions of acute reactions to environmental substances.

Infections, whether bacterial, viral, or fungal, are acidifying. The pH factor is the most pervasive factor occurring in both acute maladaptive reactions and chronic degenerative disease substance reactives (brief systemic and longer term local).

Unfortunately, the specialty of allergy settled on the evidence of antibody reactions as providing the believable reactions to environmental substances and for some years disregarded and tended to disbelieve any type of reactions that did not manifest antibodies. If the allergy specialty had taken the acid pH-hypoxia factors as the central reason for reactions, allergy would have been the specialty that contributed most of all specialties to the advancement of medicine.

The acidity is local where the symptoms develop and may not necessarily be reflected by an assessment of the blood pH. Morning (AM) blood pH is not a reliable indication of the degree of disease and acidity-hypoxia in local symptom areas. The systemic evidence (blood pH), if and when present, after a maladaptive reaction, classically becomes corrected in two to three hours.

In an acid medium, molecular oxygen becomes reduced and no longer has oxidative value. Since molecular oxygen is necessary for biological energy production in humans, the development of hypoxia in an acid medium is central to the acute and chronic disease process.

The Physiological Effects of Positive and Negative Magnetic Fields

According to many researchers, negative magnetic fields seem to affect all the metabolic processes involved in growth, healing, immune defense, nonimmune microorganism defense, and detoxification. The following chart was prepared by William H. Philpott, M.D. and is based on his clinical observations of the effects that positive and negative magnetic fields have upon living organisms.

Biological Response to Antistressful Negative Static Magnetic Fields	Biological Repsonse to Stressful Positive Static Magnetic Fields
pH normalzing	Acid producing
Oxygenating	Oxygen deficit producing
Resolves cellular edema	Evokes cellular edema
Usually reduces symptoms	Often evokes or exacerbates existing symptoms
Can relieve addictive withdrawal symptoms	Stress evokes endorphin production and symptoms can therefore be addicting
Inhibits microorganism replication	Accelerates microorganism replication
Biologically normalizing	Biologically disorganizing
Governs rest, relaxation, and sleep	Governs wakefulness and action
Evokes anabolic hormone production-- melatonin and growth hormone	Evokes catabolic hormone production inhibits anabolic hormone production
Counters and processes metabolically- produced toxins out of the body	Produces toxic end products of metabo- lism and does not counter or process these toxins out of the body
Cancels out free radicals	Produces free radicals

The Role of Exogenous Energy Sources

Physiologists figure that no more than 70% of human biological life energy comes from the food digested. Energy is required to process this food and therefore, the net gain of energy is about 70%. Where does the 30% of exogenous energy come from and what can we do to enhance this 30%?

Humans live in a magnetic field and become ill if not in a magnetic field. Astronauts are provided an artificial magnetic field to prevent illness. A fluid passing through the friction of a magnetic field produces electromotive energy. This is used industrially. Blood flowing in the human body, which is flowing through the earth's magnetic field in which the human lives, will provide the production of some electromotive energy. This energy production can be enhanced by placing a magnet over the heart. Using the negative magnetic pole also keeps the cellular elements properly magnetically poled so they do not stick together. Also, oxygen and water are paramagnetic and can carry this magnetic field to the entire body through the blood circulation.

The earth's magnetic field is waning and therefore humans are living in a magnetic deficient environment. This can be corrected by sleeping on a negative poled magnetic bed pad and/or with the head in a negative magnetic field.

Wearing the negative pole of a magnet on the heart will help correct the magnetic deficient environment.

Any treatment of the body with a magnetic field will to some degree have a systemic energy increase since the oxygen and water passing through the magnetic field become magnetized, which then goes to the entire body.

It is of interest to note that insects and sharks obtain 90% of their energy from exogenous sources whereas humans receive only 30% of their energy from exogenous sources.

The Case of Pat Sos

Pat Sos[29] reported on the Internet, "I've found remarkable relief by doing my own research — and I'm willing to share information with you. I've used magnetic therapy for the past two years and two months and now am walking without the wheelchair and crutches, no more expensive office visits (up to $700 a visit), no more steroid shots, and [I've gone] from 12 pills a day to just one a night.

"I wake up refreshed with more energy and less stiffness. I've lost cartilage in the spine, neck and shoulders and the doctors totally gave up when they told me I had Fibromyalgia/Fibrositis and Rheumatoid Arthritis.

"I can now drive for the first time in years.

"Self-use magnetic therapy may not be for everyone — but has certainly helped me. I've saved money not only on the doctor bills and medications, but don't have to have someone pick me out of the bed each morning! The swellings in my joints are gone.

"I may add that some people may experience increased pain during the first few days or weeks of using magnetic therapy, but this is commonly known as the 'healing crisis,' caused by the body dispersing toxic buildups. (See The Herxheimer Effect," http://www.arthritistrust.org.)

"I have letters of appreciation from all over the country telling of how others have improved their lives by using this easy therapy at home."

Dr. Bob Arnot adds, "It's not pain relief alone that has doctors excited. Biomagnetic therapy may be reversing the degeneration of joints and promoting the growth of new cartilage."[29]

This author advises that you cannot afford to overlook magnetic therapy. Go to Amazon.com and you can order Philpott's 740 page book. It's easy to read and provides treatment protocols for almost everything.

Massage Therapy

In a study performed at the Touch Research Institute, Miami School of

Medicine, in 1994, 30 adults were divided into three groups, one given massage for 30 minutes twice a week for 5 weeks; the second group received an electrical impulse treatment applied to the painful area (TENS) for the same time period; the third group received dummy TENS over the same time period.

Assessing results based on changes in fibromyalgic tender points, all groups had a reduction in pain, "but only those receiving massage reported decreases in pain, fatigue, stiffness and improvements in the quality of sleep."[8]

Massage researcher Richard Van Why reported that Sweden's Karolinska Institute completed studies using a vibrational massage of 100 to 200 cycles per second applied to pain points for 15 to 30 minutes. These studies showed great relief in pain. Dr. Chaitow states that "using the hands to vibrate the skin, by using firm pressure plus a rapid vibration, appears to produce the same benefits without causing any negative effects."[8]

In another Swedish study, 21 out of 26 patients "noted improvement after massage; after repeated treatment, patients experienced reduced pain, plus a gradual decline in the increase in blood myoglobin concentration."[31]

Mineral Infrared Therapy

Dr. Tsu-Tsair Chi has reported on an infrared ceramic-coated device that has beneficial effects in strengthening the immune system, decreasing pain, unblocking lymph channels, increasing circulation, and providing lacking trace elements.[126]

Neural and Intraneural Injections

Intraneural Injections

Dr. Paul K. Pybus serendipitously but independently discovered the effect of intraneural injections on certain key neuromata in the treatment of Osteoarthritis and Rheumatoid Disease, as based on theories taught by Roger Wyburn-Mason thirty years earlier.

The Arthritis Trust of America feels that his booklet, *Intraneural Injections* is a must for all forms of arthritits and arthritis-like pain, and that the use of designated intraneural injections decreases the time to wellness, regardless of what other modalities are used on the patient. (See Intraneural Injections at Amazon.com.)

Englishman Roger Wyburn-Mason, M.D., Ph.D., nerve specialist, was the first to describe the causation principle of joint damage from tender nerve locations, sometimes called "trigger points," in arthritis and arthritis-like pain.

South African Dr. Paul K. Pybus, his former house physician, learned to implement in clinical practice Wyburn-Mason's theories of intraneural injections, successfully using his discoveries for more than 20 years.

American Keith McElroy, M.D. independently discovered the same principles, and applied them to his patients, also for many years.

Dr. Paul K. Pybus and Gus J. Prosch, Jr., M.D. explored additional key "trigger points," until it became clear to them that a virtual one-to-one correspondence existed between painful neuroma and acupuncture points -- but not always so.

Dr. I.H.J. Bourne, a friend of both Dr. Roger Wyburn-Mason and Dr. Paul Pybus, also developed the use of intraneural injections which he published as "Musculoskeletal Disorders: Local Injection Therapy."

Specialists in musculoskeletal pain have long used area-wide; i.e., non-specific "trigger points," intraneural injections and intra-articular injections, as well as nerve blocks to relieve pain. In other words, although their medical territory was not really inclusive, they unwittingly discovered some of the same points for patient pain relief. At the suggestion of Dr. Curt Maxwell, we recommend the W.B. Saunders book, *Atlas of Pain Management Injection Techniques* by Steven D. Waldman, M.D., J.D. as an excellent supplementary book. (It is very convenient for doctors who are into reimbursement via insurance, as it gives the insurance code that is acceptable for each of the injections.) The artwork is excellent, and there can be no doubt as to how to inject in the various parts of the body. The text is quite appropriate, giving not only the how, but also contra-indications, et. al.

Of most importance, however, for more than 50 years American Harry H. Philbert, M.D. independently developed the use of intraneural injections which he called "Specific Injection Therapy," covering many of the same aspects as the publications reported above. *The Anatomy of Pain: Specific Injection Therapy*, is a well-done report of Dr. Philbert's research.

Dr. Philbert's work will shock most medical practitioners, as he claims through his techniques alone to have improved the lot of many painful patients, and, in particular, has easily cured bronchial asthma, and other conditions, including some coronary problems. We're very sorry to report that we don't know where to purchase this extremely fine book.

As sensitive nerve trigger points are often the source of pain, Neural and Intraneural Injections can often relieve the pain, and sometimes result in per-manent relief.

In the Huenke Neural Therapy, an anesthetic such as procaine or lidocaine is injected into nerve sites of the autonomic (independent) nervous system, acupuncture points, scars, glands, and other tissues. Through the pathways of the autonomic nervous system, energy to cells short-circuit the disease or injury and serves to regulate biological energy.

Although an individual injection can relieve pain, it is a series of injections that follow along a key physiological pattern that serves to provide the most relief.

Premised on the idea that illness begins when the normal flow of biological energy is disrupted, Neural Therapy seeks to release these energy blockages, and sometimes the results are quite spectacular, providing an almost instantaneous "miracle" cure.

Any part of the body that has been damaged or traumatized can cause these energy blockages, thus the injections may follow old wounds, surgical scars, past body blows, "stored" illnesses, and so forth.

Neural therapy can also assist in unblocking the lymph system.

Conditions that normally respond to Neural Therapy include arthritis, allergies, back pain, and about thirty more.

Dietrich Klinghardt, M.D., Ph.D. of Santa Fe, New Mexico, adds that "In my experience, between one and six treatments, given twice weekly, are all that's needed."

Intraneural Injections
The Nature of Joint Pain

Reconstructive therapy normalizes and balances the structure of the whole body through the tightening up of lax or torn ligaments and tendons powered by muscles. Keeping in mind that it is the ligaments and tendons, together with bones, that provides the body's overall structural shape, nonetheless prolonged unevenly applied muscles contribute to osteoarthritis and rheumatoid arthritis by creating prolonged, uneven stress at specific joints. This prolonged, uneven application of muscle power applied through perfectly normal tendons and ligaments has its ultimate source-causation from specific nerve centers that usually lie very close to the skin. (See "Sclerotherapy, Proliferative Therapy, Reconstructive Therapy: Treatment of First Choice for Osteoarthritis and for Other Athritic-like Pain," http://www.arthritistrust.org.)

English Professor Roger Wyburn-Mason, M.D., Ph.D., nerve specialist, demonstrated more than 50 years ago that the source-causation of joint pain in both osteoarthritis and rheumatoid arthritis began with disturbances in the cells of nerve centers called "ganglia." Although "source" of pain may be the same, causation may differ in different disease state.

South African Dr. Paul Pybus, surgeon and acupuncturist, demonstrated that these disturbed nerve ganglia usually corresponded to traditional acupuncture points normally found along the nerve paths of uninsulated nerve fibers that lay close to the surface of the skin (called unmyelinated C-fibers), unlike the deeper, insulated fibers that carried larger electric signals throughout the body. One key nerve center -- ganglion -- for example, is protected by the bony protubance at the base of the small finger of each hand at the back of the wrist. At the base of that bump, on the little finger side, will be found a special nerve from which signals flow to specific parts of the fingers. If that nerve is pressed and there is no pain it is not inflamed or creating problems with the fingers under its "command." However, if pain is experienced when pressing that point, then one has found a key source of finger joint pain.

Another major nerve center, or ganglion, is found at the elbow's "crazy bone," also somewhat protected by a bony protrubance. Between the elbow and the wrist, between the two bony sites described, there are many smaller nerve centers that also may be painful when pressed. Each one of these when inflammed and painful on touch is the source-causation of pain which appears to stem from the joints, and which is traditionally called "joint pain."

Dr. Paul Pybus and Gus Prosch, Jr., M.D. traced out a large number of these especially critical nerve centers throughout the body as related to both osteoarthritis and rheumatoid arthritis, as well as other forms of rheumatoid diseases such as ankylosing spondilitis, fibromyalgia, and so on. In almost every instance the center of joint disturbance follows known acupuncture points.

The Method of Applying Intraneural Injections

Gus J. Prosch, Jr., M.D. taught the theory and practice of Intraneural Injections techniques to more than 600 physicians on osteoarthritis, rheumatoid arthritis and as many as 79 other rheumatoid and other diseases. He has also treated more than 12,000 patients using the techniques of Intraneural Injections. (See *Intraneural Injections: Intraneural Injections for Rheumatoid Arthritis and Osteoarthritis and The Control of Pain in aRthritis of the Knee*, Dr. Paul K. Pybus Amazon.com)

Knowing the underlying structure of the nerve network leading to each joint, the physician presses with his thumb, finger, or pen (palpates) over points of expected tenderness. The tender points will be known by observing the patient wince, or the patient will respond in some manner saying, "Right there! It hurts."

Each tender point is marked with a skin pencil.

Next a mixture of anaesthetic and a form of cortisone that does not act systemically -- that is, throughout the body -- is injected into the disturbed nerve site. We do not, of course, condone the use of cortisone for systemic use (throughout the body), or for use in the traditionally applied manner to dampen the symptoms of pain. However, studies show that the form of cortisone described here acts only locally, thus is called "depot" for the fact that when "deposited" in one site it stays there, and only slowly dissipates without any of the dangerous consequences that normally accompany the traditional use of cortisone. (The mixture may be 1-1/2% procaine with a small amount of Depo-Steroid such as Triamcinolone Hexacetonide).

This small bleb inserted at the nerve-ganglia found to be tender will immediately halt the pain.

The reason the Fibroymyalgia patient reports aches from head to toe is that certain key pain points in the body are tender to touch: knee pain, back pain, shoulder, arm and hand pain.

Dr. Philibent uses only Lidocaine HCl for effective treatment.

Curt Maxwell, D.C., N.M.D. of Algondones, Mexico (across the border from Yuma, Az) has also found that the Depo-Steroid mixture is unnecessary and, indeed, receives a large number of Americans who, by word of mouth, have been referred to him and this effective treatment of "Intraneural injections," "Injection Therapy," or "Specific Injection Therapy."

The Case of Marie Ray, R.N.

Marie Ray, full time Registered Nurse, wrote for Dr. Maxwell the following:

"The pain was stealing my life! Here I was, a new snowbird just retired and ready to enjoy the freedom. Instead I found myself living a vicious cycle of fatigue due to the inability to sleep, caused by the excruciating hip pain that would come in the night and frustration because I couldn't walk long enough or far enough to enjoy anything. I couldn't participate in the dances or sight-seeing or anything active because my legs ached so badly!

"Yet inactivity was my worst enemy, and as soon as I sat down to relax, my muscles would stiffen up and the pain would set in worse. So I would move around, walk a little then sit again. This was the retirement I had looked forward to for years?

"Several years ago I suffered a bad back injury and the spasms and pain just slowly increased even though I had tried everything: acupuncture, massage, chiropractic, water exercises, stretching, pills, nothing helped for very long. then one day I was introduced to Dr. Maxwell. He had made the mistake of saying he wished he had a big challenge, then I walked in the door and he got his wish! By now there was hardly a place between my waist and my knees where I could stand to be touched much less stuck by a needle! "Hot spots" were everywhere, some no more than 1/2 inch apart. Every nerve was inflamed, every muscle in constant spasm and I was miserable, at the end of my rope. But, not being a quitter I was willing to try anything.

"Today, 3 months and 8 sometimes painful treatments later, I sleep all night, the fatigue is gone, the hot spots are gone and the nerves in my legs and hips no longer scream with every step. The spasms are slowly relaxing and now it is up to me to take the responsibility for the rest of my recovery, do the necssary correct stretching 3-4 times a day, exercise and take the supplements pre-scribed.

"Thanks to the knowledge, caring and persistence of Dr. Maxwell my life is mine again. Also my heartfelt thanks to his wife Esperanza for her encourage-ment, understanding and gentle loving support during some very difficult times.

"I will be back next year, but I seriously doubt it will need to be as a patient because this is where my search ended and my new lease on life started! I will be eternally grateful to Dr. and Mrs. Maxwell!"

A year later, Marie Ray wrote:

"I'm back, but not for any treatment. Since first seeing Dr. Maxwell … I have come so far! … No more hip, leg, or back pain! I dance, I work and thank God, I sleep! I travel alone and do what I please! Life is great.

"I feel great and I owe it all to Dr. Maxwell!"

Nutritional Therapy

Additional helpful supplements to those mentioned earlier may include vitamin B12 (intramuscular injections) repeated daily, calcium, magnesium, proteolytic enzymes between meals, vitamin C with bioflavonoids.[4]

Physical Therapy

Often relief for Bursitis can be achieved by following the directions of Agatha Thrash, M.D. and Calvin Thrash, M.D..[49]

• Avoid injury to joints that are especially vulnerable to Bursitis. A strain, a direct blow, the stress of overweight, unusual shoulder or knee motions such as from painting, swimming, and lifting heavy objects at arm's length, may precipitate Bursitis.

• Allergies and infections elsewhere in the body may bring on Bursitis. Live at a high level of health to avoid Bursitis.

• Do not allow excessive fatigue to develop while doing an unusual motion to which you are unaccustomed. When heavy objects must be taken in the hand for some distance, the best position is in front of one, using both hands to hold the object somewhat like a tray.

• Do not allow chilling of the extremities, particularly the shoulders, which are especially vulnerable at night. Be careful to wear warm sleepwear.

• Never begin heavy work until you have 'warmed up' by doing some light work.

• Use these treatments for Bursitis:

A. Heat applications may relieve pain.

B. Ice packs to the painful area, especially in the acute phase, may relieve pain. Keep the ice on for about five to seven minutes. Remove for one minute, and repeat three times.

C. Place the patient in an upper-half body pack, as in bronchitis — [In bronchitis, spread a plastic on the bed and place on it two double steam packs crosswise over the area where the patient will lie, from neck to waistline. Cover well with towels and have the patient lie down. For comfort, elevate the head and flex the knees high over a bolster. Fold a single steam pack, wrap it in a towel, and lay it over the patient's upper chest for 15 minutes. Remove the last one, and after using a vigorous cold friction rub on the hot area, apply a fresh hot pack — making sure the upper edge is above the shoulders. Place a single steam pack over the shoulder. Cover the pack with plastic to retain heat, keeping steam out of the patient's face, and leave it in place and hot for 20 minutes. Replace with another hot one (no cold), then a third, covering a period of one hour. Finish with a shower, sponge bath, or alcohol rub.] Repeat this treatment daily until the pain is gone. Early mild cases clear up in a day or two. Chronic or severe ones may require three weeks or more.

D. Hot and cold compresses are sometimes helpful in relieving the inflammation. Use three minutes of hot compresses as hot as can be tolerated, followed immediately by twenty seconds of ice water compresses. Repeat four times. Give the treatment three or four times daily.

E. Do not use deep massage as it may increase inflammation. Superficial stroking will be beneficial.

F. A short period, 1-3 days,of complete rest for the part may decrease inflammation. A sling may be worn with much comfort. Do not prolong the period of inactivity, as a stiff joint may result.

G. Exercises: Use after any hot or cold treatment:

1. Wall-walking exercise: Face the wall at arm's length and lean into your hands placed against the wall. Starting slightly above the level of the waist, walk hand over hand as high as you can reach without pain. As you make progress, reach higher each time before pain or tightness stops you. Repeat the exercise four times daily.

2. A small pulley rigged up over the head with a two to five pound weight attached is helpful after the acute phase is over. Pull the arm down by the side and let the weight pull the arm over the head. Start with five to ten pulls and work up to 50 three times a day.

3. A bicycle wheel with a small handle attached and mounted shoulder-high can be used to good advantage to get a good range of motion of the shoulder, avoiding a 'frozen shoulder.'[49]

Qigong for Arthritis

Pronounced "Chi Gong" chinese energy work, or "Qigong" has exploded into Western awareness during the past twenty years.

Roger Jahnke, O.M.D.,[55] Santa Barbarba, California, has had dozens of patients with Fibromyalgia. "We feel that Fibromyalgia is an overall degenerative disorder that is not really a muscle disease, . . . that the symptoms are not the cause.

"We found through regular massage, acupuncture and Qigong, that most cases will improve very dramatically."

The Case of Crystal Starburger

Crystal had a very severe case of Fibromyalgia, and had gone off work using workman's compensation. She was "stagnating in her house and dissatisfied with numerous doctors who had given her a whole array of medications, all of which did nothing."

Dr. Jahnke reports that, "Our strategy was to help her understand Fibromyalgia, that it is caused and then perpetuated by the person's choices — their personal choices.

"In this case it seemed acupuncture was somewhat helpful, but the shift in life style and practice of Qigong was the most important parts of Crystal's wellness, because she discontinued the acupuncture treatments and kept improving. What I believe she found most important was that she learned to meditate into gentle body movement types of exercises, which is what Qigong is.

"Crystal began having steady improvement to the extent that she returned to work, basically completely cured.

"Most people we've seen who've had this disorder work too hard, they don't rest efficiently, and they build up a deficiency in stimulating the body's ability to eliminate toxic substances. They build up toxicity.

"We see that when people began to meditate, chew their food more slowly, do gentle exercise on a regular basis — and that means never doing aggressive exercise — and when they do gentle massage of the hand, foot, and ear, and do deep breathing exercises — this contributes to producing less metabolic byproducts that are toxic, and to removing more toxic materials."[55]
****

See Roger Jahnke, O.M.D., books, *Qigong: Awakening and Mastering the Medicine Within*, *The Self Applied Health Enhancement Methods*; tape, *Deeper Relaxation for Self Healing*, Health Action, 243 Pebble Beach, Santa Barbara, CA 93117; Dr. Yang Jwing-Ming, *Arthritis — The Chinese Way of Healing and Prevention, The Root of Chinese Chi Kung: The Secrets of Chi Kung Training*, YMAA Publication Center, 38 Hyde Park Avenue, Jamaica Plain, Massachusetts 02130.
****

Master Jwing-Ming Yang

Jwing-Ming Yang,[39] who has written a series of books clearly explaining this ancient Chinese knowledge, was born in Taiwan, Republic of China in 1946. He started his Gongfu/Wushu (Kung Fu/Wushu) training at age of fifteen under a Shaolin White Crane master Cheng Ging Gsao. He later studied Yang Style Taijiquan (or Tai Chi Chuan) under Master Kao Tao for three years. From Master Kao Tao, Dr. Yang learned the barehand Yang style form, Taiji breathing, and Qi (Chi) exercises.

When Jwing-Ming Yang was eighteen-years-of-age he entered Tamkang College in Taipei Hsien to study physics, and while there he studied Shaolin Long Fist (Chang Quan) with Master Li Mao-Ching, and advanced his Taiji training with Master Li. Later he practiced and studied together with a classmate, Mr. Wilson Chen "who was learning Taijiquan with one of the most famous masters in Taipei, Master Zhang Xiang-San."[39]

Dr. Yang completed his master's degree in physics at the National Taiwan University, served in the Chinese Air Force, returned to Tamkang College to teach physics, and to continue his study under Master Li Mao-Ching. In 1974 Dr. Yang studied mechanical engineering at Purdue University (United States) where he founded a Chinese Kung Fu Research club and also taught accredited courses in Taijiquan, also to be awarded his Ph.D. in 1978.

In Houston, TX, while working for Texas Instruments, Dr. Yang founded

Yang's Shaolin Kung Fu Academy.

In Boston, where he moved, Dr. Yang founded Yang's Martial Arts Academy (YMAA), later giving up his engineering career to research, write and teach in Boston.

Besides extensive travel to many foreign countries, Dr. Yang has written twenty-four books and published twenty-one videotapes on Qigong and martial arts. There is little doubt that Dr. Yang can authoritatively blend western thinking with health/martial arts discoveries that are far, far older than Western civilization itself.

<u>What is Qi (Chi)?</u>

In Dr. Yang's description of historical Chinese views, Qi "is the energy or natural force which fills the universe," of which there are three general types: heavenly Qi, the forces which heavenly bodies exert on the earth, Earth Qi, which absorbs the Heaven Qi, and human Qi which is influenced by the other two.

The pervasive themes are "balance, harmony and interactive influence."

Perhaps one reason why ancient Chinese healing lore has taken so long to penetrate Western civilizations' thick skins is that emphasis is not upon solving a disease problem, but rather on restoring the balancing energy of vital life forces, the Qi forces, from which health then flows; that is, the result is that disease states disappear when the life force is rebalanced.

In Western terms, Qi is the body's bioelectricity whose strength, of course, is subject to "balance, harmony and interactive influence." This bioelectric field can be measured and manipulated through Qigong exercises, spiritual contemplation, emotional rebalancing, and thought. There is also a glimmer of hope that modern technology can also enhance the electromagnetic field effects of one's own bioelectric activity.

<u>Historical Background of Qigong</u>

Dr. Yang divides the history of Chinese Qigong into four periods:

• 2690 B.C. to 1154 B.C.: While acupuncture was not mentioned in Chinese writings dating back to 1766-1154 B.C., the *Jia Gu Wen* (*Oracle-Bone Scripture*), there is evidence that "stone probes" (Bian Shi) were used during the reign of the Yellow emperor from 2690-2590 B.C., and that these probes were being used to adjust Qi circulation.

• Before 1122 B.C. to Han Dynasty 206 B.C.: *Yi Jing* (*Book of Changes*) was introduced before 1122 B.C., lasting until Buddhism and its meditation methods were imported from India, bringing Qigong practice and meditation into the second period, the religious Qigong era.

• 1122 B.C. to 934 B.C.: Breathing techniques were mentioned in Lao Zi's (Li Er) Classic on the *Virtue of the Dao* (*Tao Te Ching*), stressing the way to obtain health was to "concentrate on Qi and achieve softness."

• 770 B.C. to 221 B.C.: *Historical Record* (*Shi Ji*) described more complete methods of breath training.

• 300 B.C. (approximately) Zhuang Zi, Daoist philosopher, described the relationship between health and the breath in *Nan Hua Jing*.

• 206 B.C. to 502-557 A.D.: Discovery that Qigong could be used for martial purposes. Thousands-of-years-old Buddhism imported to China from India. Buddhism became popular through emperor's influence. Since much of the training was aimed at obtaining Buddhahood, the principles were kept secret. Zhang Dao-Ling combined traditional Daoist principles with Buddhism, creating a religion called Dao Jiao, combining Daoism with Buddhism.

Tibetian training systems and methods were also imported, and absorbed. "Contemporary documents and Qigong styles show clearly that religious practitioners trained their Qi to a much deeper level, working with many internal functions of the body, and strove to obtain control of their bodies, minds, and spirits with the goal of escaping from the cycle of reincarnation."

During the 3rd century, Hua Tuo, a famous physician, used acupuncture for anesthesia in surgery.

Daoist Jun Qian used the movements of animals to create the *Wu Qin Xi* (*Five Animal Sports*), "teaching people how to increase their Qi circulation through specific movements."

Physician Ge Hong used his mind "to lead and increase Qi."

During the period of 420 to 581 A.D. Tao Hong-Jing compiled "*Yang Shen Yan Ming Lu* (*Records of Nourishing the Body and Extending Life*) which showed many Qigong techniques."

From 220 B.C. to 220 A.D. there are written references to (1) breathing to increase Qi circulation by Bian Que in *Classic on Disorders* (*Nan Jing*); (2) the use of Qi and accupuncture to maintain good Qi flow by Zhang Zhong-Jing in *Jing Kui Yao Lue* (*Prescriptions from the Golden Chamber*); (3) the relationship of nature's forces and Qi by Wei Bo-Yang in *Zhou Yi Can Tong Qi* (*A Comparative Study of the Zhou* [dynasty] *Book of Changes*).

• 502-557 A.D. to 1911: Martial Qigong styles were created based upon Buddhist and Daoist Qigong. A Buddhist monk, Da Mo, former Indian prince, was invited to China to preach Buddhism. As the emperor did not like the monk, Dao Mo withdrew into a Shaolin Temple where he found the priests were weak and sickly. After nine years of seclusion, and consideration of the problem, he wrote two classics: *Yi Jin Jing* (*Muscle/Tendon Changing Classic)* and *Xi Sui Jing* (*Marrow/Brain Washing Classic*).

According to Dr. Yang, "the *Muscle/Tendon Changing Classic* taught the priests how to gain health and change their physical bodies from weak to strong.

"The *Marrow/Brain Washing Classic* taught the priests how to use Qi to clean the bone marrow and strengthen the blood and immune system, as well as how to energize the brain and attain enlightenment."

66

The *Marrow/Brain Washing Classic* training was held in secret, passed only to a few disciples each generation, because it was harder to understand and practice.

After the priests used the muscle/tendon changing exercises, "they found that not only did they improve their health, but they also greatly increased their strength. When this training was integrated into the martial arts forms, it increased the effectiveness of their techniques.

"The Shaolin priests also created five animal styles of Gonfu which imitated the way different animals fight. The animals imitated were the tiger, leopard, dragon, snake, and crane.

• 581 A.D. to 907 A.D.: Chao Yuan-Fang compiled the *Zhu Bing Yuan Hou Lun* (*Thesis on the Origins and Symptoms of Various Diseases*) listing 260 different ways to increase the flow of Qi.

Sun Si-Mao described the method of "leading" Qi — directing Qi to specific body parts — in *Qian Jin Fang* (*Thousand Gold Prescriptions*) and also described Six Sounds to regulate Qi internal organs, the Six Sounds having already been in use by Buddhists and Daoists.

Sun Si-Mao introduced his Lao Zi's Massage Techniques in *Wai Tai Mi Yao* (*The Extra Important Secret*) which discussed use of breathing and herbal therapies for disorders of Qi circulation.

• 960 A.D. to 1279 A.D.: "Chang San-Feng is believed to have created Taijiquan (or Tai Chi Chuan). Taiji followed a different approach in its use of Qigong than did Shaolin. While Shaolin emphasized Wai Dan (External Elixir) Qigong exercises, Taiji emphasized Nei Dan (Internal Elixir) Qigong training. "External, here, means the limbs, as opposed to the torso which includes all vital organs. Internally means in the body instead of in the limbs." After thousands of years of searching for elixer, a hypothetical life-prolonging substance, elixer was found inside the body. "In other words, if you want to prolong your life, you must find the elixer in your body, and then learn to protect and nourish it."

" . . . In 1026 A.D. the famous brass man of acupuncture was designed and built by Dr. Wang Wei-Yi." Before that time there was much disagreement about acupuncture theory, principles and techniques. Dr. Wang Wei-Yi also wrote *Tong Ren Yu Xue Zhen Jiu Tu* (*Illustration of the Brass Man Acupuncture and Moxibustion*).

Dr. Wang Wei-Yi explained for the first time the relationship of the 12 organs and the 12 Qi channels, also systematically organizing acupuncture theory and principles. As the success of acupuncture spread, Dr. Wang also dissected the bodies of prisoners and added more information to the advance of Qigong and Chinese medicine, describing the circulation of Qi in the body.

From 1127-1279 A.D. Marshal Yue Fei created several internal Qigong exercises and martial arts. It is believed that he created the set of exercises applicable to medicine known as the "Eight Pieces of Brocade," to improve the health of soldiers. Marshal Yue Fei "is also known as the creator of the internal martial style Xing Yi."

Eagle style martial artists also claim that Yue Fei was the creator of their style.

• 960 A.D. to 1368 A.D.: Zhang An-Dao wrote *Yang Shen Jue* (*Life Nourishing Secrets*) discussing several Qigong practices.

Zhang Zi-He wrote *Ru Men Shi Shi* (*The Confucian Point of View*) describing "the use of Qigong to cure external injuries such as cuts and bruises."

In *Lan Shi Mi Cang* (*Secret Libary of the Orchid Room*), Li Guo describes Qigong and herbal remedies for internal disorders.

Ge Zhi Yu Lun (*A Further Thesis of Complete Study*), written by Zhu Dan-Xi, provides a theoretical explanation for the use of Qigong in curing disease.

From 1279 A.D. until 1911 A.D. many other Qigong styles were founded, and many documents related to Qigong were published.

• 1911 onward: "Chinese Qigong training was mixed with Qigong practices from India, Japan, and many other countries." Qigong practice entered a new era, as China became known by the remainder of the world. What had been taught secretly either by martial artists, or by religious organizations, found its way into the stream of the world's consciousness, and also people were able to compare Chinese Qigong to similar developments in India, Japan, Korea and the Middle East.

Categories of Qigong

Qigong practices aim at rebalancing Qi bioelectrical energy, maintaining its strong flow, maintaining health, healing when necessary, for spiritual enlightenment, and for fighting.

Theory of Qigong

• During the past twenty years, western medicine has gradually begun to accept the existence of Qi and its circulation in the human body. It is also a growing trend to accept that disease is an imbalance in the electrical flow of the body, such a concept corresponding rather well with the concept of Qi as developed several thousand years ago.

• Being the case, then all disease states can be conquered, or changed, by changing the flow of bioelectrical energy.[39]

• According to Roger Jahnke, O.M.D., "Qi, in China, is not thought of as an energy the way we relate to it. The best definition that I've come up with is 'naturally occurring internal self-healing resource.' By this definition you're including physical as well as electromagnetic as well as chemicals, as well as whatever performs the functions."[55]

• According to Dr. Yang,[39] "In order to use Qigong to maintain and improve your health you must know that there is Qi in your body, and you must understand how it circulates and what you can do to insure that the circulation is smooth and strong."

• There are two divisions of Qi: Managing Qi (Ying Qi), sometimes called "Nutritive Qi," and Guardian Qi (Wei Qi).

Managing Qi is energy that has been sent to the organs so that you can function. Guardian Qi has been sent to the surface of the body to protect you from negative influences such as the cold.

To keep yourself healthy, you must learn to manage these two types of Qi.

• Corresponding to the now well-known acupuncture meridians, the human body has twelve major channels through which Qi circulates. There are also eight vessels that store Qi. The twelve channels are like twelve electric lines, with capacitors for excess electrical storage located throughout the body.

• "When the Qi in the eight reservoirs is full and strong, the Qi in the rivers is strong and will be regulated efficiently. When stagnation occurs in any of these twelve channels or rivers, the Qi which flows to the body's extremities and to the internal organs will be abnormal, and illness may develop."

• Apparently the function of the reservoirs are to replenish the flow in the twelve major channels that interconnect all bodily organs whenever Qi becomes low in various bodily parts.

• Factors necessary for proper creation and conduction of bioelectrical energy are (1) natural energy received by interaction with electromagnetic fields; (2) food and air; (3) the way we think, as thought creates the electromagnetic force that leads to Qi to energize emotion which energizes appropriate muscles to action; (4) exercise.

So, in Taiji Qigong, "the mind and the movements are two major sources of electromotive force."

• According to Dr. Yang, "Before you start your Qigong training, you must first understand the three treasures of life — Jing (essence), Qi (internal energy), and Shen (spirit) — as well as their relationship. If you lack this understanding, you are missing the root of Qigong training, as well as the basic idea of Qigong theory. The main goals of Qigong training are to learn how to retain your Jing (essence), strengthen and smooth your Qi flow, and enlighten your Shen (spirit). To reach these goals you must learn how to regulate the body (Tiao Shen), regulate the Qi (Tiao Qi), and regulate the Shen (Tiao Shen)."

• "Regulating the body includes understanding how to find and build the root of the body, as well as the root of the individual forms you are practicing. To build a firm root, you must know how to keep your center, how to balance your body, and most important of all, how to relax so that the Qi can flow."

• "Regulating the mind involves learning how to keep your mind calm, peaceful, and centered, so that you can judge situations objectively and lead Qi to the desired places. The mind is the main key to success in Qigong practice. "

• "To regulate your breathing, you must learn how to breathe so that your breathing and your mind mutually correspond and cooperate. When you breathe this way, your mind will be able to attain peace more quickly, and therefore concentrate more easily on leading the Qi."

• "Regulating the Qi is one of the ultimate goals of Qigong practice. In order to regulate your Qi effectively you must first have regulated your body, mind, and breathing. Only then will your mind be clear enough to sense how the Qi is distributed in your body, and understand how to adjust it."

For a complete description and details, see *Qigong for Arthritis* by Dr. Yang Jwing Ming.

The Chinese Approach to Arthritis

Chinese physicians evalute the imbalances of Qi, or what Westerners call "bioelectricity," as well as by noting the actual physical symptoms. According to ancient Chinese lore, Qi becomes unbalanced before a disease or sickness appears. If the unbalance is not corrected, then physical damage results, because every cell in the body requires Qi to survive, and without its normal abundance, the cell functions improperly, or dies.

Chinese physicians, and their patients, try to correct the imbalance before it results in destruction to the cells, joints, and systems.

Chinese medicine does not differentiate between different forms of arthritis, as does the West, because they are all caused by an imbalance in the body's bioelectrical energy, which, in any case, must be corrected for the body to repair itself as far as it can do so after damage has resulted.

Restricting negative enviromental exposures as well as proper diet are considered important in Chinese medicine, although the latter is often enhanced with a vast storage of data related to the use of herbs.

Dr. Yang lists these ways as means for treating arthritis:

• Prevent arthritis from happening, or from getting worse.

• Massage, when properly done, can improve Qi circulation in the joint area.

• Acupuncture can temporarily halt pain and also increase Qi circulation. Western physicians have also shown that it can strengthen the immune system.

• Herbal remedies are used to alleviate pain, increase Qi circulation, help healing of injuries, and speed up healing.

• Cavity Press (Dian Xue) is a "method of using the fingertips (especially the thumb tip) to press acupuncture cavities and certain other points (pressure points) on the body in order to manipulate the Qi circulation."

While it may take years to learn to use acupuncture properly, according to Dr. Jang Jwing-Ming, Cavity Press can be learned quickly and requires no equipment.

"In Cavity Press, stagnant Qi deep in the joint is led to the surface. This improves the Qi circulation in the joint area, and considerably reduces the pain. The use of cavity press to speed up the healing of injured joints is very common in the Chinese martial arts."

• Qigong exercises for arthritis have the main purpose of rebuilding the strength of the joint by improving Qi circulation. As long as there is a proper supply of Qi at the joints, they can be repaired and, in some cases, even be rebuilt.

"Practicing Qigong can not only heal arthritis or joint injury and rebuild the joint, it is also known to be very effective in strengthening the internal organs. Many illnesses, including some forms of arthritis, stem from abnormally functioning internal organs."

According to Roger Jahnke, O.M.D.,[39] "Qigong accelerates oxygen distribution in the body at a time when your muscles are not rapidly using it as they would be in aerobics or running. This enables cells to begin their repair work.

"Second, there is a tremendous benefit to the immune system. Qigong shifts the body into a state where the autonomic nervous system moves toward the parasympathetic-sympathetic balance, which then supports and enhances the activities of the immune system.

"Third, Qigong helps to turn on the body's 'garbage disposal system' known as the lymph [sysem], thereby eliminating toxins, metabolites, and pathogenic factors from the tissues." (See "Lymph Detoxification" and "Lymph Drainage," http://www.arthritistrust.org.")

With a healthy flow of Qi circulation, internal organs will be healthy, the immune system will be strengthened, and the spirit will be at peace.

Reconstructive Therapy

Reconstructive Therapy can be very successful in alleviating, or completely solving various forms of Bursitis or Fibromyalgia. Whenever tendons or ligaments are stretched or torn, the body compensates by producing stress or pain in another part of the body. Reconstructive therapy tightens up tendons and ligaments, thus eliminating pain. (See "Sclerotherapy, Proliferative Therapy, Reconstructive Therapy: Treatment of First Choice for Osteoarthritis and for Other Arthritic-like Pain," http://www.arthritistrust.org.)

The Case of Alberta Hardwick

Alberta Hardwick, 42-years-of-age, a pharmacist, had diffuse body aches, and even required a neck brace to get through the day. When Ross A. Hauser, M.D.,[52] Caring Medical & Rehabilitation Services of Oak Park, Illinois conducted a physical examination, he found "exquisitely tender" Fibromyalgia points over the 18 characteristic positions. Other symptoms included numbness, stomach pain, stiffness, pain in the arms, temporomandibular joint (TMJ: jaw/hinge joint), legs, lower back, neck, shoulders, and shoulder blades, and Alberta also suffered from difficulty in sleeping.

Alberta had been hospitalized for pain, and also had had several courses of physical therapy as well as acupuncture, none of which had granted her any significant relief.

Dr. Hauser adminstered prolotherapy (called sclerotherapy, proliferative therapy, or reconstructive therapy) to her back, neck, shoulder blades, arms and jaw-hinge joint.

Within two months, Alberta felt overall better, her numbness less, and she no longer needed her neck brace. Dr. Hauser repeated the treatment.

Four months later Alberta was doing much better, and sleeping better. Her low back was good except after washing the floor, a great improvement. Before treatments, she could barely bend over let alone wash the floor.

Prolotherapy was done in the involved areas, and no further treatments have been needed. Alberta is doing well and enjoying life again.

The Case of Blanche Berry

Blanche Berry, 42-year-old beautician, had suffered significant hip pain. Ross A. Hauser, M.D. found her to have Bursitis (left trochantric).

Prolotherapy injections were done around the left hip, and when she returned a month later she reported that swimming and walking were a lot better.

Prolotherapy was done again on the left hip, and a month later Blanche noticed that she no longer had the hip pain. She stands and bends as a hairdresser about 28 hours per week, and has been doing great since.

Reflexology

Reflexology was introduced into America by William Fitzgerald, M.D., a laryngologist at St. Francis Hospital in Connecticut, and later developed by Eunice Ingham, a physiotherapist.[4]

Dr. Fitzgerald based his work out of an earlier European process called "zone therapy," discovering that he could induce numbness and alleviate certain symptoms by applying finger pressure to specific points on the hands and mouth.[4]

Eunice Ingham mapped organ reflexes on the feet and developed techniques for creating a stimulating effect in those areas.

Reflexologists feel that a precise pressure applied to the correct points on the foot will correspond with an influence on internal organs and glands in the body. "Nerve endings in the feet have extensive interconnection through the spinal cord and brain to all areas of the body," writes Ray Wunderlich, M.D. of Florida.[4]

Reflexology is practiced by nearly twenty-five thousand certified practitioners around the world, and more than 50,000 people have taken reflexology seminars.[4]

Appyling reflexology techniques to the foot in the right location can stimulate the adrenal glands, releasing natural cortico-steroids, which can relieve
72

the pain and inflammation of various forms of arthritis, according to Laura Norman, author of *Feet First: A Guide to Foot Reflexology*.[20][2]

Each session should last 15 to 20 minutes and be done once a day.[20]

Stress Relief

All dietary factors can be related to degree of stress. Stimulants and free-radical generators, such as caffeine, alcohol and tobacco, need to be as low as possible, preferably zero, according to Leon Chaitow, D.O.[8]

The muscles need to release their tensions, which might be achieved through massage, stretching, exercise, hydrotherapy, or better nutrition.

Hydrotherapy, a neutral temperature bath, can profoundly relax the nervous system.[8]

Using proper breathing methods can also help, as this leads to better circulation and oxygenation, and reduces feelings of anxiety.

Bodywork and massage treatment — various forms — and stretching movements — yoga, T'ai chi, or muscle energy-type releases — are almost certainly necessary if the problems are chronic.

Leon Chaitow, D.O. outlines in his book, *Fibromyalgia: What Causes It, How It Feels, and What to Do About It,* specific techniques that each patient can use to handle tender trigger points and relieve muscle strain. *[8]*

If one has trouble sleeping, several "natural" substances can be used. The amino-acid tryptophan, of course, is the best. Dr. Chaitow also suggests the use of chlorella and other blue-green algae. Drinking a mixture of one of these in the evening will provide as much tryptophan as would a few grams of full-spectrum amino acid powder or capsule.

Melatonin from plant sources, 2 to 3 grams before bedtime, will help induce sleep and relieve depression.

Arginine and ornithine, two other amino acids, may be taken for a period of two or three months, only, with a rest period before starting again to prevent imbalances of amino-acid body chemistry. These two are growth hormone precursors, and should never be taken by anyone who has not reached their physical maturity.

Ornithine is preferred with 2 grams taken in the morning and evening.

When arginine is taken, the dosage is double, or 4 grams taken in the morning and evening.

The amino acid DL-phenylalanine, 2 to 3 grams daily in divided doses between meals, has been shown to have painkilling potential.[8]

Always supplement the amino acids with vitamins A, C and E.[8]

There are many books and processes for reducing stress, and except for general principles outlined *"Stress"* (see http://www.arthritistrust.org) this foundation, each person must search, discover and try-out for themselves that mode of life-style which best fits their own unique personality and physical condition.

Early research with Rheumatoid Arthritis and "Rheumatism," involved staphylococcus and streptococcus killed organisms injected as antigens, the successful results thus strongly supporting the infectious nature of Rheumatoid Arthritis. As many forms of Rheumatoid Disease, or related dysfunctions, seem to have an infectious and/or allergenic component, such as Ankylosing Spondilitis, Candidiasis, Crohn's disease, Fibrositis, Fibromyalgia, food allergies, rhinitis, and so on, this form of protection may be not just all-inclusive, but also cheap and all-important.

Injecting known, specific allergens or antigens into the cistern (base of teat) of a cow just prior to calving produces protective substances that are curative.

This form of treatment has been shown to be effective with a wide variety of ailments including Rheumatoid Disease, Rheumatism, coughing, respiratory problems, sore throat, skin conditions, acne blemishes, upset stomach, cold and flu, diarrhea, and impetigo. (See *Universal Oral Vaccine*, http://www.arthritistrust.org.)

References

1. *The Merck Manual of Diagnosis and Therapy*, 16th Edition, Merck, Sharp & Dohme Research Laboratories, Division of Merck & Co., Inc., Rahway, N.J., 1992.

2. *Textbook of Internal Medicine,* J.B. Lippincott Company, East Washington Square, Philadelphia, PA 19105, 1989.

3. Paul Davidson, M.D., *Are You Sure It's Arthritis?* Macmillan Publishing Company, 866 Third Avenue, New York, NY, 10022, 1985.

4. Burton Goldberg Group, *Alternative Medicine: The Definitive Guide*, Future Medicine Publishing Co., Puyallup, WA, 1994.

5. John Marion Ellis, M.D., *Free of Pain*, National Headquarters, Natural Food Associates, PO Box 210, Atlanta, Texas 75551, 1988.

6. William H. Philpott, M.D., Bio-Electro-Magnetics Institute, Institutional Review Board, 17171 S.E. 29, Choctaw, OK 73020; *The Magic of Magnetic Healing* at Amazon.com.

7. Roberta Wilson, *Aromatherapy for Vibrant Health & Beauty*, Avery Publishing Group, Garden City Park, New York, 1995.

8. Leon Chaitow, D.O., *Fibromyalgia: What Causes It, How It Feels, and What to Do About It*, Thorsons, 1160 Battery Street, San Francisco, CA 94111-1213, 1995.

9. Alan R. Gaby, M.D., "Nutrient of the Month: Potassium-Magnesium Aspartate: A Special Supplement for Tired People," Nutrition & Healing, c/o Publishers Mgt. Corp., PO Box 84909, Phoenix, AZ, 85071, October 1995.

10. Alan H. Pressman, D.C., Ph.D., "Metabolic Toxicity and Neuromuscular Pain, Joint Disorders, and Fibromyalgia," *Townsend Letter for Doc-*

tors & Patients, 911 Tyler St., Port Townsend, WA 98368-6541, November 1995, p. 80-81.

11. *Journal of Internal Medicine*, 235:199, March 1994.

12. *Journal of Rheumatology*, 20:344, February 1993.

13. Martin Zucker, "Boswellia: An Ancient Herb Combats Arthritis," *The Natural Way*, June/July 1995.

14. Raul Vergini, M.D., *Magnesium Chloride Hexahydrate Therapy*, Supplement to the Art of Getting Well, The Arthritis Fund/The Rheumatoid Disease Foundation, http://www.arthritistrust.org; also published in *Townsend Letter for Doctors*, 911 Tyler Street, Port Townsend, WA 98368, November 1992, p. 992.

15. Nan Kathyrn Fuchs, Ph.D., "Calcium Controversy," *The Natural Way*, April/May 1995, p. 12-13.

16. Alan Gaby, M.D., "Capsaicin Treatment for Fibrmyalgia," *Townsend Letter for Doctors & Patients*, 911 Tyler St., Port Townsend, WA 98368-6541, October 1995, p. 19.

17. Robert C. Atkins, M.D., *Dr. Atkins Health Revolution: How Complementary Medicine Can Extend Your Life*, Houghton Mifflin Company, Boston, MA 1988.

18. Murray C. Sokoloff, M.D., "Foreward," *Arthritis Relief at Your Fingertips*, by Michael Reed Gach, Warner Books, New York, New York, 1989, p. viii.

19. Michael Reed Gach, "Arthritis and Nonarticular Rheumatism," *Acupressure's Potent Points: A Guide to Self-Care for Common Ailments*, Batam Books, 1990.

20. Laura Norman, Thomas Cowan, Feet First: A Guide to Foot Reflexology, Simon & Shuster, New York, New York.

21. M. Penny Levin, Ph.D., Acupuncture.Com; E-mail: AcuCom@Aol.com.

22. Personal interview with Warren Levin, M.D.

23. Personal letter from Richard A. Kunin, M.D.

24. David Squires, "Fibromyalgia — David's Story," *A Resource Catalogue*, To Your Health, Inc., 11809 Nightingale Circle, Fountain Hills, Arizona 85268.

25. Kate Lorig, R.N., Dr. P.H., James F. Fries, M.D., *The Arthritis Helpbook*, Addison-Wesley Publishing Company, Third Edition, 1990, 23.

26. Dr. Tsu-Tsair, N.M.D., Ph.D., *Mineral Infrared Therapy*, Chi's Enterprises, Inc., 5465 E. Estate Ridge Rd., Anaheim, CA 92807, 1993.

27. J.B. Chapman, Ph.D., J.W. Cogswell, M.D.; revised D.S. Rawson, M.A., *Dr. Schuessler's Biochemistry*, Thorsons Publishing Group, Rochester, Vermont, 1986.

28. Leslie N. Johnston, D.V.M., "Fibromyalgia — Rheumatoid Arthritis,"

Townsend Letter for Doctors, 911 Tyler St., Port Townsend, WA 98368-6541 August/September 1995, p. 93.

29. Internet: #: 60299 S2/Holistic Medicine; 26 October 1994 08:33:57; Sb: #59746- Rheumatoid Arthritis; Fm Pat Sos 75051, 1601; To: Barbara Havlena 74001, 2545; refers to "Medical Magnetism— A Healing Force Coming of Age, Martin Zucker, *Lets Live* magazine, March 1993; "Magnetic therapy KO's Arthritis Agony," Jim O'Brien, *Your Health* magazine, April 6, 1993; "The Surprising Healing Power of Magnets," Jane Heimlich, *What Your Doctor won't Tell You*, April 1993; Dr. Bob Arnot, "Stop the Pain" series, *CBS This Morning*, February 9, 1993.

30. Sherry A. Rogers, M.D., "Real Relief From Fibromyalgia," *Women's Health Letter*, Vol. IV, No. 9, September 1995.

31. Harald Gaier, N.D., D.O. H.P., "Fibromyalgia," Alternatives, September 1995, p. 9; reported from *Br Homeopath J.* 1986; 75(3): 142-7; *Br Med J*, 1992; 305:1249-52; *Scandinavian J Rheumatol*, 1986; 15 (2): 174-8.

32. Dr. Andrew Lockie, *The Family Guide to Homeopathy*, Fireside, Rockefeller Center, 1230 Avenue of the Americas, New York, New York 10020, 1989.

33. Guy E. Abraham, M.D., Jorge D. Flechas, M.D., M.PH., "Management of Fibromyalgia: Rationale for the Use of Magnesium and Malic Acid," *Journal of Nutritional Medicine* (1992) 3, 49-59, p. 49.

34. Dr. Christine Northrup, "Overcoming Fibromyalgia," *Health Wisdom for Women*, Vol. 2, No. 11, 711 Montrose Road, Potomac, MD 20854-3394, May 1995.

35. Zoltan Rona, M.D., M.Sc., "Help For Fibromyalgia," *Alive*, #154, p. 23.

36. "We Spoke to Bonnie Prudden About Defrocking Fibromyalgia," The Planned Parenthood women's Health Letter, May 1995, Vol. 2, No. 3.

37. Debbie Carson, "Kombucha Tea," (reporting on Gunther W. Frank, *Kobucha*) in *Trans*, PO Box 121851, Nashville, TN 37212, Summer 1995, p. 14; Can be contacted at (615) 889-4701; also contact Elizabeth Baker, author of *The Uncook Book*, and others, PO Box 149, Indianola, WA 98342 (206) 297-2271.

38. Anne Ineson, *Cell Tech's Global Vision Hope, Health & Freedom*, 660 Bremen Road, Waldoboro, Maine 04572; (207) 832-5366; (800) 927-2527, independent distributor for Cell Tech.

39. Jwing-Ming Yang, *Arthritis — The Chinese Way of Healing and Prevention,* YMAA Publication Center, Yang's Martial Arts Association (YMAA), 38 Hyde Park Avenue, Jamaica Plain, Massachusetts 02130, 1991.

40. "An Anti-Inflammatory Aid: Feverfew" Julie Nowak, *Health Points*, TyH Publications, 11809 Nightingale Circle, Fountain Hills, AZ 85268, 1995.

41. "About Fibromyalgia Syndrome," *Health Points*, TyH Publicaitons, 11809 Nightingale Circle, Fountain Hills, AZ 85268, 1995.

42. "Arthritis," *Alternative Medicine Digest*, Future Medicine Publishing Co., Issue 8, 5009 Pacific Highway East, Suite 6, Fife, WA 98424,1995.

43. Roger Jahnke, O.M.D., *Alternative Medicine Digest*, Future Medicine Publishing Co., Issue 9, 5009 Pacific Highway East, Suite 6, Fife, WA 98424,1995.

44. Joseph G. Hattersley, July 14, 1995 to Burton Goldberg.

45. Personal communication with Harold Buttram, M.D.

46. Correspondence with Jorge A. Meneses, PO Box 2001, Lenox Hill Station, New York, NY 10021.

47. K.M. Lucero, "The Electro-Acuscope/Myopulse System: Impedance-Monitoring Microamperage Electrotherapy for Tissue Repair," *Rehab Management: The Journal of Therpay and Rehabilitation*, Volume 4, Number 3, April/May 1991.

48. Personal letter from Jerry Fisher, president, Electro-Medical Incorporated.

49. Agatha Thrash, M.D., Calvin Thrash, M.D., *Home Remedies*, Thrash Publications, Rt. 1, Box 273, Seale, Alabama 36875.

50. Dava Sobel, Arthur C. Klein, "Bee Venom," *Arthritis: What Works*, St. Martin's Press, 175 Fifth Avenue, New York, NY 10010, 1989; Also see *Alternative Medicine Digest*, Future Medicine Publishing, Inc., 5009 Pacific Highway East, Suite 6, Fife, WA 98424.

51. Personal correspondence with Paul A. Goldberg, M.P.H., D.C.

52. Personal correspondence from Ross A. Hauser, M.D.

53. Personal interview with Hector Solorzano del Rio, M.D., Ph.D., D.Sc.

54. *Desert Arthritis Pak*^{TM} *Instructional Booklet: Immunotherapy, Nature's Way of Fighting Arthritis,* Arthritis in Remission Ltd., A Division of B & G Marketing Group, Inc., 1232 Drexel Ct., N.E., Grand Rapid, MI 49505; (800)-624-6353.

55. Interview with Roger Jahnke, O.M.D.

56. "Intestinal Sluggishness," *Alternative Medicine Digest*, Issue 10, Future Medicine Publishing, Inc., 5009 Pacific Highway East, Suite 6, Fife, Washington 98424, January 1996, p. 24.

57. Sunshine Company, 223 W. 3325 N., North Ogden, Utah, 84414; (801) 782-5552.

58. Peter Smrz, M.D., "Complementary Treatment of Post- and Parainfectious Rheumatoid Disorders," *Biological Therapy*, Vol. XIV, No. 1, 1996, p. 156.

59. Adeena Robinson, *Iron: A Double Edged Sword*, Informasearch, 1995.

60. R. Paul St. Amand, M.D., *Fibromyalgia*, August 1996.

www.ingramcontent.com/pod-product-compliance
Lightning Source LLC
Chambersburg PA
CBHW070916180526
45168CB00005B/2033